The Easy Yoga Exercise Book

By The Same Author

True Yoga
Yoga For The Mind

The Easy Yoga Exercise Book

YOGI WILLIAM ZORN

PELHAM BOOKS

First published in Great Britain by
PELHAM BOOKS LTD
52 Bedford Square
London, W.C.1
May 1971
Second Impression September 1971
Third Impression May 1976

ISBN 0 7207 0423 5

Photoset in Great Britain by
Filmtype Services Limited, Scarborough, England,
in 689 Univers 9/11 point. Printed by
Hollen Street Press Ltd at Slough and
bound by Dorstel Press at Harlow, Essex

CONTENTS

ACKNOWLEDGEMENTS

I wish to thank Carol Preston for posing so gracefully for the Yoga postures. She has been an enthusiastic student of Hatha Yoga for several years and, as the pictures show, it certainly has done her no harm.

George Jantscher was the artist with the camera.

Drawings by Andrew Bokor.

ILLUSTRATIONS

INTRODUCTION

If you would like to try some Yoga because you have heard this can do you a great deal of good, but the thought of having to stand on your head frightens you, and the idea of having to fold your legs into some impossible knot puts you off altogether, then this is the book for you. Neither the headstand nor the lotus posture will be mentioned here. Instead, you will find an abundance of simple physical exercises and easy Yoga postures which you will be able to practise without any previous experience. There are indeed many advanced and extremely difficult techniques in the field of physical Yoga, or Hatha Yoga as it is called, but this fact should not be a deterrent. Many are the exercises and Yoga postures which you can perform to your great benefit, even if you have not done anything energetic for years and feel as stiff as can be. Yoga need not be complicated in order to be beneficial.

There is no denying that to-day medical science has come a long way. Organs are being transplanted successfully, and cures for many diseases once thought incurable have been found. However, a pill to extend youth and prolong life has, as far as I am aware, not yet been developed. That glowing feeling of well-being which comes from physical fitness and radiant health cannot be obtained from a bottle. In the absence of an 'elixir of youth,' right living is still the best guarantee for good health and longevity, and sufficient exercise forms an integral part of the right way of life. Movement is just as important to the body as air, water and food.

Many of the minor illnesses and irritating physical complaints which beset mankind are the results of unnatural living and mental anxieties. The leading of a healthy life will soon have a marked effect upon physique as well as upon psyche. Proper exercise will stimulate the circulation of blood throughout the blood vessels and tissues, form the muscles and help to make excess fat disappear. The breathing action is improved, and heart and lungs kept healthy. Listlessness and tiredness become things of the past. After only a little while energy and fitness thought lost forever flow back into the body, and life can again be enjoyed to the full. Even sleep is more restful.

The ancient science of Yoga provides us with a system for exercising every part of the body, and for learning to control the unruly mind. There is no age limit for the practice of Yoga. It is just when you get older that the need for proper exercise becomes more urgent. When you are young you play sport and are physically more active in general, but as you get older you become occupied with other things. Sitting at a desk, driving your car, and watching TV from the depth of an armchair, you are not living as actively as you should. Your body is meant to move — walking, running, climbing. By not moving enough your body becomes old before its time. Yoga does much to delay old age. It helps to keep the joints and the spine supple, improves the digestive powers of the body, and ensures good elimination. Insufficient bowel action is one of the prime causes of premature ageing and illness, as it causes chronic poisoning of the system. In Yoga, much attention is paid to the abdominal region. Also, the glands are made to work better, which is why the practice of Yoga has a rejuvenating effect on the whole body.

You don't need any special equipment when you exercise the Yoga way. You can practise in the privacy of your room or garden. You do need a sensible approach. Yoga should never be forced, and at no time should you overreach yourself. If you are told in the text to 'try to touch your toes' and you can only get down as far as your knees, well and good. With practice you'll get there in the end; Rome was not built in a day. It is advisable to set aside some time each day for your exercises. When? Well, the time which suits you best is the best time. However, you should always try to have an empty stomach — exercising immediately after a meal is not only uncomfortable, it can be dangerous. Try to put all things from your mind, and devote the time entirely to your well-being.

Clothing should always be light and comfortable, and the room in which you practise should be well-ventilated, so that when you breathe in deeply you inhale nothing but wonderful fresh air. Should you at first get dizzy from deep breathing, just rest a little. Your system has to adjust itself to the large oxygen intake.

A warning is in order. *Should there be something physically wrong with you, or should you even suspect that there is, consult your physician before you start.* For the rest, use common sense.

People with high blood pressure should avoid exercises which cause the blood to flow to the head — those in which the head is down — or postures where the legs are raised. The same goes for people with heart trouble, who should not do anything too strenuous.

In the case of a slipped disc, bending in the wrong direction will aggravate the trouble, and the utmost care should be taken. Those with an ulcer should not bring too much pressure to bear on the abdominal region. Any exercise which causes pain or discomfort should be discontinued, and strenuous exercises avoided. Remember — don't worry too much; few things are worth ruining your health for.

Pregnant women can do light exercise, but would be wise first to consult their doctors. They should avoid causing too much pressure on the abdominal region, and not do any upward stretching.

In order to be fit and healthy, and consequently look well and feel young, you must make some effort. Therefore, exercise your way to health, and keep in good health for many years.

The introduction over, get ready to do some exercising!

1
Early Morning Routine

If you were to get out of bed in the morning, stand up and try to touch your ankles or your toes while keeping the legs straight, you would find it a near-impossible task, even if normally this feat would cause you no trouble whatsoever. The body is very stiff after a night's rest; there is some movement during sleep, but it is far from sufficient to keep the joints and the spine in a flexible state. This makes us realise that we would be completely immobilised if we were to go without any form of exercise. Conversely, the more we exercise the fitter, more supple and healthier we will be.

So take it easy first thing in the morning. The body should be limbered up only gently. Certainly you do not start with Yoga postures, even though you may have performed those postures quite easily the previous day. Therefore, here is a ten-minute morning routine which you will find most useful and enjoyable. It is an excellent way to start the day.

Stretching
Before you do anything else, stretch yourself luxuriously several times while you take a few deep breaths. This surely is a wonderful feeling! Stretch yourself a few more times if you wish.

Deep Breathing
Now for a deep-breathing exercise. Breathing is one of the most important functions for maintaining life. Most people just don't breathe deeply enough. They use perhaps only one-third of the full capacity of their lungs, and this is a great pity. Breathing fresh air brings oxygen to all the cells of the body. Millions upon millions of living cells make up the human body, and each of these needs oxygen. The body cannot function properly if the cells do not get the required supply of oxygen. Many people would be a lot healthier and have much more vitality if only they breathed deeply enough. Therefore, let us start the programme with some deep breathing.

Stand up straight with the legs together and the arms down beside the body. As you commence to breathe in, slowly bring the arms up sideways and continue to breathe in till the arms are above the head with the fingers touching. Breathe out evenly as you slowly bring the arms down the same way. Repeat the deep-breathing exercise as often as you wish. The effect is not just that of a breathing exercise, as you are already loosening up various muscles in a mild way.

9

Cleansing Breath

Normally one should always breathe in and out through the nose, but here you exhale through the mouth. Stand with the legs wide apart and reach with the arms high above the head as you breathe in deeply through the nose. Throw the air out through the mouth, making the sound 'Ha' as you bend forward, keeping the legs straight, hanging the head down and allowing the arms to swing loosely. Don't reach down at all, as the spine is still very stiff. Force the breath out with the 'Ha' sound a few more times, keeping the head down, till the last bit of stale air has been expelled from the lungs. Repeat this cleansing breath several times.

Loosening up Shoulders

You are ready for some light physical exercises. First you can loosen up the chest and shoulder muscles by circling both shoulders slowly in the same direction. After a little while, roll the shoulders the opposite way.

Upward Stretching

For a good stretching exercise, stand with the arms high above the head, look up and try to reach higher with each hand in turn. Reach ever higher before finally bringing the arms down. Repeat the exercise while standing on your toes, and reach higher still.

Twisting

Next give the spine some horizontal movement. Stand up straight with the legs together, breathe in deeply as you bring the arms high above the head and lock the fingers with the palms facing up. Hold breath while you slowly turn the trunk to the left as far as you can. Continue to hold your breath as you come back and then slowly turn the trunk to the right as far as possible. Turn again to the front, and exhale as you bring the arms down.

Take a deep breath, bringing the arms high above the head, and exhale while bringing the arms down.

Circling

Stand with the legs apart and lock the hands beind the head. First describe two wide circles clockwise with the top part of the body, moving from the hips; then make two complete circles the opposite way. Take a deep breath, stretching the arms high above the head.

Ten Count Exercise

The Exercise of Ten Counts is an excellent technique to wake up properly and give the body a vigorous workout. You could put on some lively melody and swing in rhythm to the music.

Stand up straight with the legs together and the arms raised high above the head, hands held together. At Count One swing the arms back gently, and repeat this at Count Two, bringing the arms back just a little further. Hold the hands in front of the chest with the elbows kept sideways at shoulder level. At Count Three jerk the elbows back, and repeat this at Count Four, jerking the elbows back a little more.

Spread the arms sideways and swing them back at Count Five, and again at Count Six.

Count Seven and Count Eight are a repetition of Count One and Two — bring the arms high above the head and swing back twice.

Finally, bend forward and reach for the floor in a bouncing movement at Count Nine, keeping the legs straight and together. Stay down and bounce once more at Count Ten, taking care not to reach down too far.

Repeat the series as often as you wish. The first time you perform the Ten Count Exercise in the morning, go carefully. As you warm up you can put more zest into your effort. You will soon get to love the sequence, and would not miss performing it for anything.

Knee Bends

The legs must also be exercised. Nothing better for this purpose than a few deep knee bends slowly executed. Place the hands on the hips, or lock them behind the head. Raise yourself on your toes, then slowly bend the knees till you are squatting on your heels. Come up equally slowly and repeat the exercise several times. Try to stay on your toes throughout. Afterwards give the legs a little shake and take a deep breath as you stretch the arms high above the head.

Push-Ups

Next for some push-ups. Lie face down on the floor and place the hands under the shoulders. As you breathe in deeply, push yourself up, keeping the body stiff and straight. Breathe out as you slowly lower yourself to the floor. Men can keep the legs straight, but the girls may, if they wish, bend the legs and push themselves up from the knees. This makes the exercise much easier, while still very useful. Keep the knees together. At first do only a few push-ups, gradually bringing up the total as you become stronger. Never exhaust yourself.

Stand up and take a few deep breaths while you stretch the arms high above your head.

You are proclaimed ready to face the day. Should you have more time, include some additional exercises in your programme at your own discretion. You will find material galore in this book.

2
The Sun Greeting

In India, the birthplace of Yoga, ancient man regarded the sun as the God of Light. He looked upon the heavenly body as the Giver of light and warmth, on whose radiant presence depended all life on earth. The devotee showed his reverence at dawn and in the evening by facing the sun and performing a series of bodily poses. This ancient ritual consisted of twelve simple postures, and as a form of exercise it has survived to this day. It is called Surya Namaskar in Sanskrit, or Sun Greeting. The execution of the twelve postures gives you an excellent combination of exercise and deep breathing. Some of the poses are traditional Yoga postures, and all are most beneficial.

The Sun Greeting affects the whole man as it works on every part of the body and has a calming influence on nerves and mind. The muscles are firmed and the circulation is improved. Heart and lungs are made strong, while the spine is kept in a flexible state. Many people suffer from constipation and poor digestion. These people will appreciate the Sun Greeting, as consistent practice thereof markedly tones up the digestive organs and improves the elimination process. Tiredness and backache are overcome. Practised in the morning on rising, a few Sun Greetings will banish sleepiness, and clear the brain. Performed in the evening before retiring, the twelve movements will calm the mind and help to overcome insomnia. Sun Greetings can be done as a preliminary to further Yoga practice, or performed on their own give you a Yoga session in miniature. The twelve poses are simplicity itself – women, children and old men alike can do Sun Greetings. The more you do the Sun Greeting, the more you will enjoy it. Regular practice through the years will help you maintain your vitality and keep your youthful looks till a ripe old age. A long life should be yours. Become therefore a sun worshipper, and diligently practise the twelve steps to fitness and health.

Now for some instructions on the subject. Wear light clothing only, and practise on a clean and firm surface; make sure you won't slip. Step on to your lawn, spread a towel, face the East and greet the rising sun. Should you be afraid the neighbours might think you have reverted to paganism, or should it be raining, you can practise in the privacy of your room. You may have to do this anyway should you live on the twenty-second floor of an apartment building in the middle of the city.

First acquaint yourself with the twelve movements and the correct order in which they are executed. Do not yet bother too much about the right breathing. Once you have become familiar with all twelve steps, make sure you are breathing correctly. In the early stages the Sun Greeting will appear to you as twelve separate movements, but after a little while these twelve movements will merge into one continuous and most enjoyable exercise.

Before you begin, stretch yourself a few times, and take a few deep breaths. At first perform only two or three Sun Greetings at a time, gradually bringing up your total. Continue the exercise as long as you enjoy it, and have a little rest afterwards.

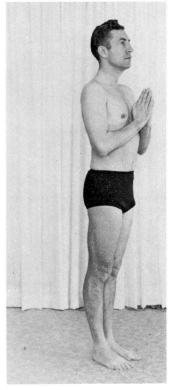

Fig. 1

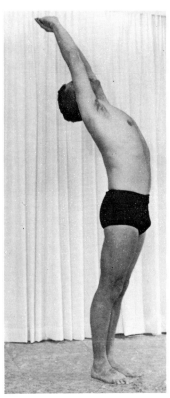

Fig. 2

Step One *(Fig. 1)*

Stand up straight with the legs together. Keep the elbows close to the body, and the hands in front of the chest in the traditional Indian greeting.

As you breathe in deeply, salute the sun (or health, life, the One). Don't hold your breath at all. Just breathe out slowly.

You have now completed the first stage, and you must admit that it was really easy.

Step Two *(Fig. 2)*

As you breathe in deeply, raise the arms high above the head and reach backwards. Get a good arch in the back and tilt the head backwards. You will find that as you reach up and lean back the chest expands and you breathe in automatically.

Hold breath and posture as long as you can comfortably do so. The exercise is good for the spine, while you will also feel a lovely pull on the abdominal muscles.

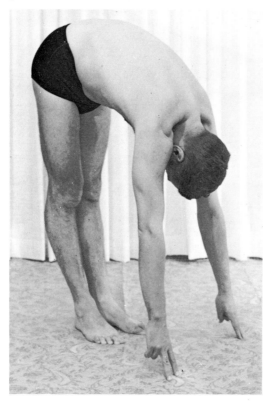

Fig. 3

Step Three *(Fig. 3)*

Bend forward and reach for the floor as you breathe out. If you cannot touch the floor, don't worry, and certainly don't strain yourself. Just go down as far as you can and bring the head towards the knees. Those who are very supple can place the fingers or the palms on the floor.

A warning is again in order — you should never strain yourself in performing the various postures, as you could easily hurt yourself. Muscles can be pulled and ligaments torn. *In over-reaching or bending or turning too much you can also damage your spine, and that of course could be disastrous. Yoga is never forced, and certainly never done in a competitive way. Everyone performs within his own physical capabilities.*

This stage of the Sun Greeting is a Yoga posture titled Padahastasana, or Hands-To-Feet Posture. Spine, back and thigh muscles all benefit. Abdominal organs are massaged, while the extra blood rushing to the head nourishes the facial tissues and tones up the thyroid and para-thyroid glands in the throat.

Keep the legs straight, even if you cannot reach the floor. You exhaled as you bent down. Inhale, keeping arms and head down, and you are ready for the next stage.

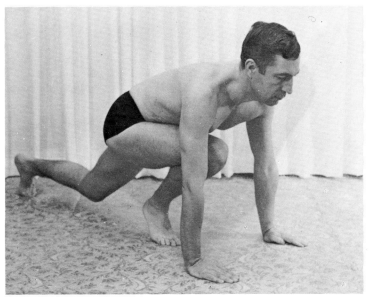

Fig. 4

Step Four *(Fig. 4)*

Here you do a number of things at once. You breathe out as you bend through the left leg and reach backwards with the right leg. The hands are flat on the floor, and the head is kept up. Don't reach too far back with the right leg; instead, have it slightly bent. The knee is only a fraction above the floor. Beginners can have the knee on the floor for support.

15

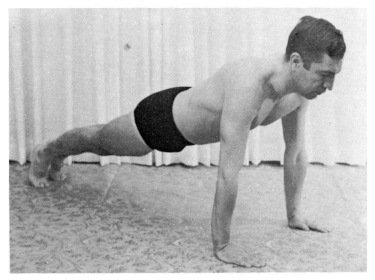

Fig. 5

Step Five *(Fig. 5)*

Now you also bring the left leg back, and simultaneously straighten both legs. Breathe in deeply as you perform this movement, and keep the body stiff and straight with the head in line with the body. Hold breath as long as you can with comfort, and as long as the muscular effort is not too much for you.

You are now in Catuspadasana, or Quadruped Posture.

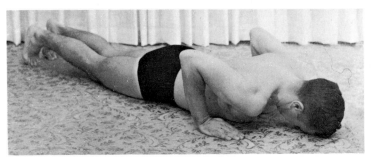

Fig. 6

Step Six *(Fig. 6)*

Slowly lower yourself to the floor as you breathe out. Coming down slowly while keeping the body stiff and straight is of course a marvellous muscular exercise for the whole body.

The hands remain in the same position alongside the chest, and the elbows are sticking up. The feet are not moved, and the forehead rests on the floor. It is in this position that you will appreciate that you should be practising on a clean surface, or on a towel.

Rest in this position should you feel the need. You are at the halfway mark, so this seems a good opportunity for a pause.

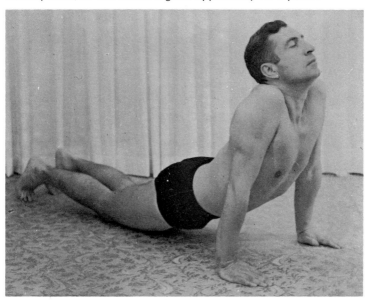

Fig. 7

Step Seven *(Fig. 7)*

The seventh step is a very popular and most beneficial Yoga position called Bhujangasana, or Cobra Posture. As you breathe in deeply, push your trunk up by straightening your arms, keeping the head up and back. The hips do not have to remain on the floor here – just straighten the arms and let the body hang between the shoulders. You will find that this will really bend your spine and give you an excellent pull on the abdomen. The benefits of this exercise are many.

The knees are on the floor. Do not change the position of the feet; keep the toes planted squarely on the floor.

Hold breath and posture as long as is comfortable. By relaxing the body completely you get that extra bend in the back and an increased pull on the abdominal muscles.

Step Eight *(Fig. 8)*

Now the body jack-knifes. The hips are brought up as high as possible while hands and feet stay in exactly the same place. Try to have the feet flat on the floor as much as you can – this will

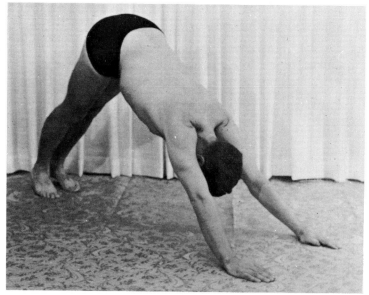

Fig. 8

produce a lovely pull on the calf muscles. The head hangs down between the shoulders.

You will discover that hands and feet should not be too far apart if you want to bring the hips up high enough. If desired, bring hands and feet a little closer, which will make the exercise easier. Should you have trouble bringing the hips up, you could leave the knees on the floor.

You breathe out while you assume this position.

Step Nine *(Fig. 9)*

In one movement, bring the right leg under the body and lift the head up. Step Nine is similar to Step Four, the only difference being that the position of the legs is reversed. This makes for a balanced exercise. In Step Four the left thigh presses against the spleen, while in the present stage the right upper leg presses against the liver.

Breathe in.

Step Ten *(Fig. 10)*

Keeping the hands flat on the floor, place the left foot close to the right and try to straighten the legs as much as you can. Be careful, and don't overdo it. You will feel the effort cause a heavy pull on the backs of the thighs. Also the muscles at the front of the thighs are strengthened. The spine is made more flexible.

When correctly executed, Step Ten is exactly the same as Step Three. The next stage will be the same as Step Two, while the final stage will be a return to Step One.

Breathe out.

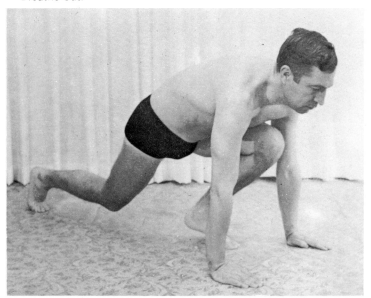

Fig. 9

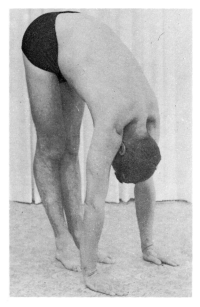

Fig. 10

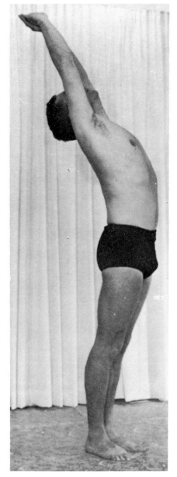

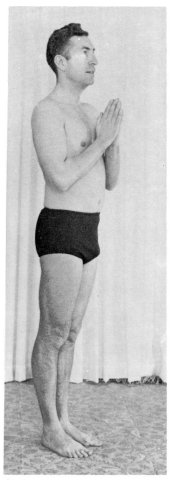

Fig. 11   Fig. 12

Step Eleven *(Fig. 11)*

Straighten up as you breathe in deeply and sweep the arms up and backwards. Hold breath and posture as long as is comfortable.

Step Twelve *(Fig. 12)*

Concluding the series, you are in the same position as when you started. You are standing up straight with the legs together, while the hands are held in the prayer position in front of the chest. Take a deep breath. Should you be a little tired, take a few deep breaths.

What you have been shown here is the slower version of Surya Namaskar. There is also a faster version, which you may like to practise once all the movements of the Sun Greeting come automatically to you. The twelve steps remain exactly the same. The tempo is brought up and the breathing alters somewhat. There is no breath retention and no holding of the poses. You breathe in as you make one movement, and out as you make the next. There is one exception, though – going from Step Three to Step Four the lungs remain empty. From then on the natural sequence continues. The movements flow into one another. The duration of the complete series executed in this manner is about thirty-three seconds.

Sun Greeting – Fast Version

Step One   —Inhale deeply and breathe out.

Step Two   —Breathe in as you sweep the arms up and back.

Step Three   —Breathe out as you bend down.

Step Four   —Keep lungs empty while bringing the right leg back.

Step Five   —Breathe in deeply as you straighten both legs.

Step Six   —Breathe out as you lower yourself to the floor. Instead of completely relaxing in this position, you keep the arm muscles contracted and the chest slightly off the floor. From there you go straight into the next position.

Step Seven   —Breathe in as you straighten the arms and bring the chest up.

Step Eight   —Breathe out as you raise the hips.

Step Nine   —Breathe in as the right leg comes under the body.

Step Ten   —Breathe out as you try to straighten both legs.

Step Eleven   —Breathe in deeply as you come up.

Step Twelve   —Breathe out and conclude the series with a deep breath.

3
Easy Yoga Postures

Here is a wide selection of Yoga postures which you can practise even if you are an absolute beginner. Postures which are too difficult have been omitted, or easier variations have been substituted.

With the bodily poses Yoga provides a method for maintaining good health and suppleness unrivalled by any other system. Although the postures help to promote a slim and shapely figure, their aim primarily is the improvement of the vital organs and the glandular and nervous systems. Much attention is paid to the suppleness of spine and joints, keeping rheumatism and arthritis at bay. Regular practice of the postures will bring relief or cure for most of the common disorders.

Before you practise the Yoga postures, do some deep breathing and a few loosening-up exercises. Attend first to the functions of bladder and bowels. In common with other forms of exercise, Yoga should never be performed on a full stomach; at least three hours should have elapsed since the last meal. Never be in a hurry when executing the postures. Be relaxed and focus the attention of your mind on the particular parts being exercised. Feel increased power and vitality stream through those parts. Never use force; some people are more supple than you, but this should not bother you in the least. If you cannot do a certain posture, just try a little — perseverance will bring quicker results than the use of force. After a few weeks of regular practice you will find yourself doing things you never thought possible. Only hold the postures as long as you can do so comfortably. If desired, you can repeat the postures you like or which you think will particularly benefit you. Have sufficient rest whenever you feel a little tired during the practice.

Fig. 13

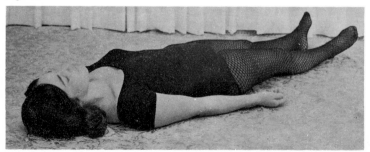

Complete Relaxation Posture *(Fig. 13)*

Perhaps the Complete Relaxation Posture appears the easiest of all Yoga postures, but its correct execution is quite an art. It is not a matter of just lying down, but of deliberately relaxing each part of the body. After the body has been brought into a state of complete relaxation, the mind is calmed. Once the pose has been mastered it brings rest and refreshment almost immediately. The posture is usually practised before and after a Yoga session. Of course it can be done at any time. People suffering from hypertension, blood pressure or heart trouble, insomnia or just plain tiredness will appreciate this ancient Yoga technique for relaxing body and mind.

Lie flat on your back and close your eyes. The arms are by your sides, a little away from the body. The hands are open, palms up. Your legs are apart, with the feet falling sideways.

First concentrate on the left leg. Breathe in deeply, at the same time tensing all the muscles in the leg. Hold breath for a moment while you also keep the muscles contracted. Suddenly you let go, breathe out and relax. Feel the leg becoming heavy and sink into the floor. After a little while, do the same with the right leg. Once that member is completely relaxed, focus your attention on the abdomen. Feel the abdomen fall down further every time you breathe out. Now you concentrate on the left arm. Breathe in deeply and tense the arm, making a fist. Hold for a moment, then breathe out and let go the muscular contraction. The arm is felt to be limp and lifeless. Next consciously relax the right arm. Then pay attention to the face; the eyes are closed, and so is the mouth; the teeth are apart, the forehead smooth and relaxed.

Deliberately slowing down the rate of breathing will calm down the activities of the mind. Yoga teaches that breathing and mental activity are very closely related. Breathe slowly, and you will calm down. You can use this knowledge to your great benefit in daily life. In times of tension, just concentrate on slow and deep breathing.

While in the Complete Relaxation Posture, abdominal breathing can be practised. As you breathe in, push the abdomen up as high as you can. The abdomen falls down again as you breathe out. Breathe deeply and calmly. Some people take a little time to master this technique; if you have trouble with it, just keep trying without forcing the issue.

Your efforts so far will have detached your mind from your other activities, from your worries and responsibilities. Relax the mind further by thinking of a beautiful and peaceful aspect of nature – a lovely sunset, a deep blue sky, or a beautiful garden. Picture this so clearly that you are completely absorbed in it. Now you are really relaxed.

Before rising from this posture, give yourself a good stretch.

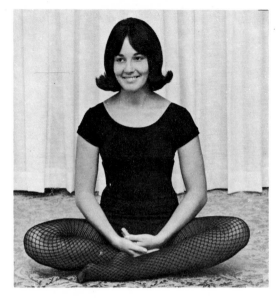

Fig. 14

Easy Posture *(Fig. 14)*

A posture which will be found most comfortable by the majority of people. The crossed feet are pulled close to the body while the hands rest in the lap, one on the other, or otherwise the arms rest on the knees. The back is kept very straight, with spine, neck and head in a straight line. Should the ankles hurt at first, you could place some soft material under the feet. It does not matter whether the knees point up in the air or are touching the floor; the main thing is that you are comfortable.

This Posture is the meditation posture par excellence, as most students can sit in this position with comfort for a considerable time. Various physical and mental exercises can be practised without distraction.

The eyes can be strengthened greatly by exercise, and this is an opportune moment. If you are wearing glasses, remove them. Keep the head still, and look up high at a point on the ceiling, focusing the eyes on it. After about five seconds, look down at a point on the floor directly in front of you. After the same time interval look up again, then down once more. Close the eyes to give them a rest, then look to the right as far as you can and focus eyes on a point on the wall there. After about five seconds, gaze at a point on your far left. After looking to right and then to the left once more, close eyes. Next slowly roll eyes in a wide circle, seeing everything. Once the circle has been completed, roll eyes in the opposite direction. Close eyes and, when you are ready, stare at the tip of the nose. Close eyes again for a rest. Stare at a point on the wall in front of you, with the eyes only half open. Conclude the eye exercises by closing the eyes and placing your palms over the eyes.

The Easy Posture is also very suitable for the practice of neck muscle exercises. Sitting up straight, slowly bring the head up and back as far as you can. Then slowly move your head forward and down as far as possible. Repeat twice more. For the next movement, carefully turn your head as far to the right as you can, and then to the left. Perform this turning movement also three times. Look up, then drop the head forward as you breathe out. The neck muscles are completely relaxed as the head drops, and the sudden pull is felt right along the spine. Repeat several times. Slowly roll the head in a wide circle, first in one direction, then in the other. Be very careful here, especially if you hear any noises from the vertebrae in the neck. At the conclusion of the series, massage the muscles by gently slapping the neck.

Breathe in deeply and sit up very straight. As you exhale, slowly bend towards the right knee. No matter if you can't reach the knee with your head. The movement should not be forced at all. Breathe in as you come up, then bend to the left knee as you exhale. Fill the lungs again as you come up, and finally bend forward and bring the head down as much as you can wile you breathe out. Remember, don't force it. You could keep the head down for a little while, keeping the lungs empty. This excellent exercise limbers up the spine and puts pressure on the abdominal organs. For constipation. Improves the digestive processes. Reduces stomach and waist.

A chin lock is applied as follows. Breathe in deeply and hold the breath as you firmly press the chin to the chest into the jugular notch. Hold breath and lock as long as you can do so without discomfort. Focus mind on the space between the eyebrows. Bring the head up as you breathe out. Improves circulation round the throat area, exercises the neck muscles, and is most beneficial to thyroid and parathyroid glands.

Yogic breathing can be practised while sitting in the Easy Posture. Some of the simpler Yogic breathing exercises are rhythmic breathing and alternate nostril breathing. For the first mentioned, breathe in for two counts, hold breath for eight counts, and breathe out in four counts. Instead of mentally counting, you can also count your pulse beats. For alternate nostril breathing you commence by inhaling deeply through the left nostril. The right nostril is closed by pressure of the fingers. Hold your breath as long as you can do so in comfort, while you focus the mind on the space between the eyebrows. The eyes are closed. Breathe out through the right nostril only, and inhale again through that nostril. Focus mind on space between eyebrows, and exhale through the left nostril, and so on.

Yogic breathing is very effective in steadying the nerves and calming the mind.

While sitting comfortably, mental exercises can be practised. An example of such an exercise — imagine that water enters the body and rises higher with every exhalation. Finally the whole body is filled with water right to the top of the head. Allow the water to remain in the body for a while and let all undesirable qualities dissolve in the water. Press the water out while you breathe in deeply, and let everything negative be flushed out with it.

Meditation falls outside the scope of this book. The subject has been discussed in the author's previous work.*

If firmly held without slumping forward, the Easy Posture strengthens back muscles and loosens the hip joints. Some people do not find it comfortable to sit in the Easy Pose; if so, sit in the Disciple Posture (*Fig. 15*), or in the Thunderbolt Pose (*Fig 16*).

People with varicose veins should not sit very long in postures where the circulation in the legs is restricted.

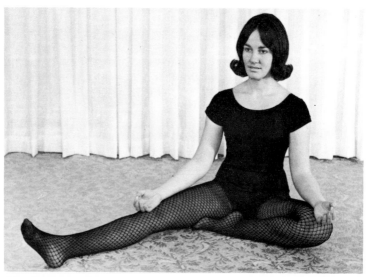

Fig. 15

Disciple Posture *(Fig. 15)*

Those who have trouble sitting cross-legged will appreciate the Disciple Posture, where only one leg is pulled to the body, while the other leg remains straight. The back is kept rigid, which makes this posture useful for strengthening the back muscles. The Disciple Posture will prove beneficial in case of backache.

The hands rest on the knees, palms up. After a while, change legs.

* *Yoga For The Mind* (Pelham Books).

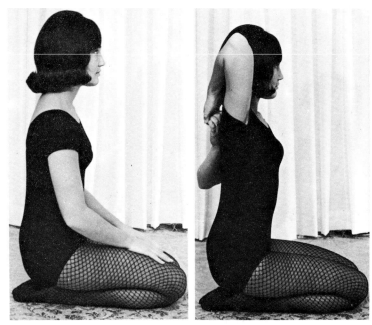

Fig. 16   *Fig. 17*

Thunderbolt Posture *(Fig. 16)*

A simple but pleasant and useful posture. Some students prefer this pose to the Easy Posture for sitting comfortably. Good for feet, ankles and knees. *Not to be practised for any length of time by people with varicose veins.*

Sit back on your heels, keeping feet and knees together. The hands rest palms down on the thighs. Back and head must be kept erect.

As in the Easy Posture, various physical and mental exercises can be practised in this position. A Yogic breathing exercise:

Inhale deeply through the nose. Hold breath and focus the mind on the space between your eyebrows. In this exercise you hold the breath for about five seconds, but no longer. Breathe out slowly and evenly through the mouth, holding your mouth as if you were whistling. You are actually making a soft, whistling sound. If you breathe out evenly, the sound is continuously at an even pitch. This exercise is called the Victorious Breath and helps to achieve good control over the breath. Yoga teaches that control over the breath leads to control over the mind.

Cow's Head Posture *(Fig. 17)*

Sit back on your heels, keeping knees and feet together. Reach over your right shoulder with your right hand, and bring your left hand

27

behind your back from below. Now try to make the fingers touch; if this presents no difficulties, lock the fingers. Don't force things, though.

Strengthens arms, chest, back and shoulder muscles, and improves the bustline.

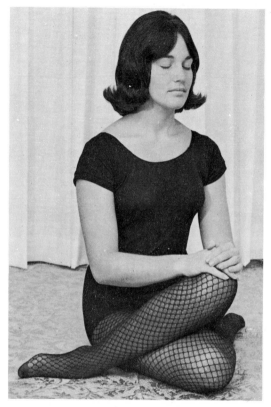

Fig. 18

Hero Posture *(Fig. 18)*

Easy for some people, difficult for others. The thighs overlap, with the right foot outside the left thigh and the left foot by the opposite side of the body. The hands are clasped around the uppermost knee. Breathe calmly, and gaze at the tip of the nose. Alternatively, close your eyes and focus the mind on the space between the eyebrows. Concentrating on this spot will be a little easier with closed eyes.

Posterior Stretching Posture *(Fig. 19)*

Sit with the legs straight and close together. Lean forward and grasp the legs just above the ankles. Breathe in deeply. As you breathe out, pull the body down with the arms, at the same time bringing the head towards the knees as close as you can. You may put some effort into it, but don't force too much. Keep the knees on the floor. Hold the posture with the lungs empty as long as you can reasonably do so, then come up slowly as you inhale. Sit up straight and take a few deep breaths.

This Yoga posture provides a marvellous stretch for the whole of the back. Bringing the head down gives added pull to the muscles and spine. The squeezing together of the abdominal section gives the internal organs a massage, helping the digestive processes and fighting constipation.

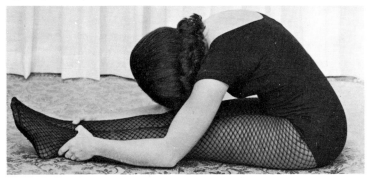

Fig. 19

Fig. 20

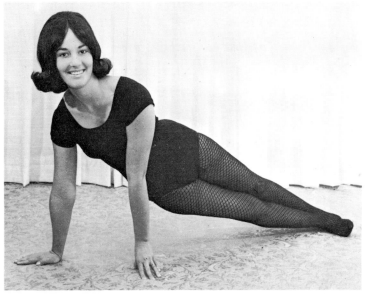

Arm-Leg Posture *(Fig. 20)*

Sit down with the legs pointing to the left, and with the hands resting on the floor to the right of the body. Slowly straighten the legs and raise the hips off the floor while still supporting yourself with both arms. If possible, the body should be brought into a straight line. Once you feel confident, bring your left arm along your side, so that you hold yourself up on the right arm only. Practise also on the other side, with the legs pointing to the right.

The Arm-Leg Posture is a good exercise for all the muscles in the body. As a more difficult variation, you can raise the free arm and leg high up in the air.

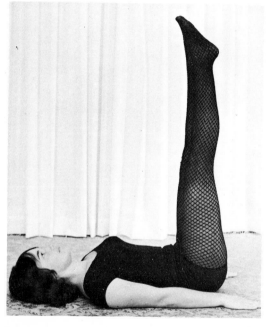

Fig. 21

Risen Leg Posture *(Fig. 21)*

Here is a posture which strengthens the leg muscles considerably, while the slow and deliberate execution of it does wonders for the abdominal muscles.

Lie on your back with the arms close to the body, palms down. As you breathe in, slowly raise the legs until they are at right angles with the body. During the ascent the legs should be kept straight for maximum results, but should this be too difficult, you may of course bend your legs a little as you bring them up. In the posture the legs should be perfectly straight and together, while the toes point to the

ceiling. Hold breath and posture as long as is comfortable, then slowly lower the legs as you breathe out.
Rest for a moment.

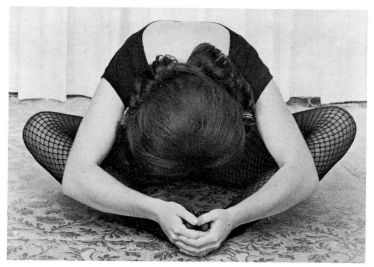

Fig. 22

Star Posture *(Fig. 22)*

Sit with the knees pointing out and the soles of the feet together. Clasp hands around the feet and inhale deeply. As you breathe out, slowly pull down, trying to bring the head towards the feet. Don't force it – it doesn't matter if you are not able to bring your head anywhere near your feet. Hold posture for as long as you can comfortably hold the lungs empty. If you can't reach your feet – and most people cannot – just let your head hang down. Breathe in as you come up slowly.

Practice of the Star Posture keeps the spine and hip joints supple, and makes childbirth easier. The digestive processes of the body are improved.

As a further exercise for hip joints and legs, you can try the following: remain seated upright, and pull the feet as close to the body as you can.

Raised Posture *(Fig. 23)*

Sit down with the legs together and straight out in front of you. The hands are placed firmly on the floor. As you breathe in deeply, raise the buttocks and right leg simultaneously off the floor. The body is then supported by the hands and the left heel. Try to keep the right leg straight and off the floor in a horizontal position, with the toes pointing away from you so that they are in line with the leg. Hold breath and posture as long as is comfortable, then come down and rest a moment. Repeat the posture, this time keeping the right foot on the floor and raising the left leg.

Strengthens arms and shoulders, and especially abdominal and thigh muscles.

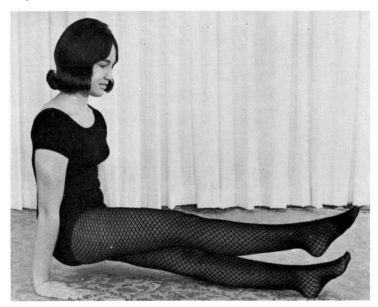

Fig. 23

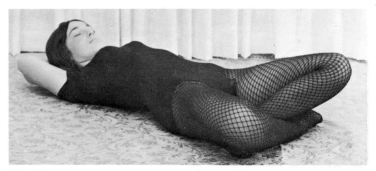

Fig. 24

Fish Posture *(Fig. 24)*

Lie on your back and pull the crossed feet close to the body. Cross the arms behind your head, placing the left hand under the right shoulder and the right hand under the left shoulder. Rest the head on the crossed arms, with eyes closed, and relax. The hip joints particularly are made loose in this posture. Beneficial in cases of constipation or menstrual troubles in women.

The Fish Posture is the ideal position for the practice of abdominal breathing, as the muscles concerned are completely relaxed.

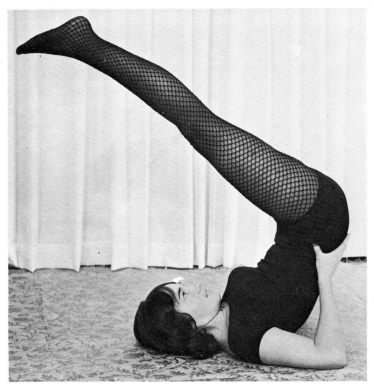

Fig. 25

Inverted Body Posture *(Fig. 25)*

In many ways Yoga is unique among the various systems for physical health. In no other field is so much attention paid to the reversing of the pull of gravity on the body. The Inverted Body Posture is a prime example. The constant pull towards the earth which slows us down and tires us, makes us want to sit or lie down, causes faces to sag and internal organs to be displaced, that force is made to work in the opposite direction by inverting the body.

Lie on your back with the legs together and the arms close along the sides. Now bend the legs and push the hips off the floor by pushing hard with the elbows. Make sure the elbows are kept close to the sides. Once you are up, place the hands under the hips for support, taking the full weight of the hips in the hands. Have the legs straight and in a forty-five degree angle. While in the posture, practise abdominal breathing, inhaling and exhaling slowly and calmly. The eyes can be closed. You will soon feel how neck, face and head are flooded with fresh blood, nourishing facial skin and stimulating the brain. If the posture becomes uncomfortable in any way, come down at once and rest for a moment.

Should you have trouble raising the hips off the floor – and some people do have trouble here – you can at first place the fists under the hips. Bring the legs up and over as far as you can, trying to keep them straight.

Regular practice of this inverted posture keeps the body in youthful condition and increases vitality. Useful in cases of thyroid deficiency and female complaints. Clears the ears and prevents wrinkling of the face. Stimulates the sex glands, aids digestion and corrects constipation. Keeps all internal organs in good working order, and eases or prevents haemorroids.

The Inverted Body Posture must be mastered before the Complete Posture can be practised.

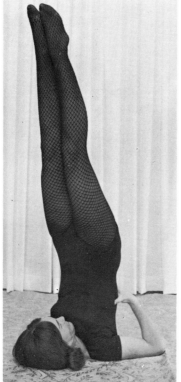

Fig. 26

Complete Posture
(Fig. 26)

As the name of this picture indicates, a great number of benefits are bestowed upon the practitioner. The complete posture is indeed one of the most beneficial postures in Yoga. The thyroid glands, which have such a bearing on a person's activity and vitality, are favourably affected. Extra blood is brought to the head and brain. Because of this extra blood supply, the face is kept young and wrinkle-free. Swollen feet and ankles as well as varicose veins are improved.

The chances of overcoming sexual debility and impotence are greatly enhanced. Prolapses are corrected. Menstrual disorders are improved, and the Complete Posture helps in cases of constipation and improves the digestive processes. The whole system is toned up and the ageing process retarded. Who would not want all this? Practise therefore with joy.

Lie flat on your back. Next bring the knees to the chest and bring the hips up. You can push off with the elbows which are kept close along your body. Place the hands in the small of the back as you straighten your legs, pointing them straight upwards. The toes also point up. Your chin is pressed to your chest.

Come out of the posture slowly and deliberately, then rest.

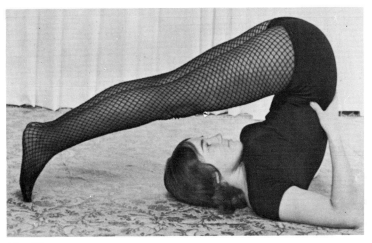

Fig. 27

Plough Posture *(Fig. 27)*

Lie on your back with the arms alongside the body. Swing the feet over the head as you push yourself up by the elbows. Gradually straighten the legs as you reach for the floor with your toes. The hands are placed in the small of the back. It does not matter at all if you can't touch the floor. *You should under no circumstances force the issue, as you can easily pull a muscle, or worse, damage your spine.* Yoga should never be forced. With practice, you will eventually get your toes to the floor. Come out of the posture slowly and gracefully, which is a good exercise in itself. Rest for a moment.

Practice of the Plough Posture makes the spine supple and tones up the thyroid and parathyroid glands in the throat. Nourishes facial tissues. Improves the digestive processes and corrects constipation.

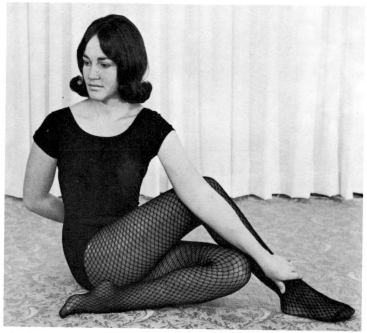

Fig. 28

Spinal Twist *(Fig. 28)*

At first sight the Spinal Twist might look a little complicated, and beginners often do seem to get their arms and legs tangled up. Therefore, concentrate!

Sit with bent legs pulled close to the right of the body. Place the right foot round the left knee. Simple enough. With the left hand you hold the right ankle. If you can, you may have the arm on the outside of the leg as shown in the illustration. Finally, place the free arm behind your back, although you may leave the free hand on the floor for support should this be necessary.

As you breathe out, turn first the head and then, slowly, the body to the right. Twist a little more while you keep the lungs empty. Don't overdo it. Turn back as you breathe in and repeat several times if you wish. Practise the posture also the other way round.

The Spinal Twist tones up kidneys, spleen and liver. The adrenal glands are invigorated, and thus the whole system benefits. The spine is kept supple, as each vertebra is involved. Corrects bad posture. Assists women in overcoming monthly cycle disorders. Tones up the reproductive organs. Fights constipation and aids the digestive processes.

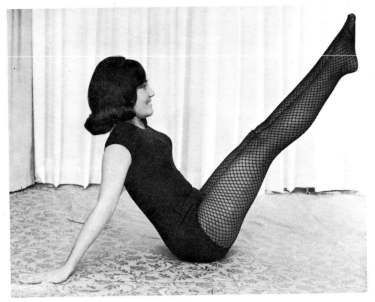

Fig. 29

Angle Posture *(Fig. 29)*

Sit with the legs drawn to the body and the feet flat on the floor. Place the hands rather wide behind you on the floor, with the fingers pointing away from you. As you breathe in deeply, raise the legs and point them up so that they are at a forty-five degree angle with the floor. As you are leaning back, the legs should be at about a ninety degree angle with the trunk. Try to keep the legs straight and hold the posture during the breath retention. Breathe out as you come down, and rest a moment.

The Angle Posture is an excellent exercise for the abdominal muscles and the legs. The solar plexus is toned up.

Archer Posture *(Fig. 30)*

Sitting with the left leg straight and the other leg bent, with your left hand get hold of toes or ankle of the left leg. Should toes or ankle be out of reach, just touch the leg with the fingers as far down as possible. With the right hand you grasp the right foot, and attempt to lift it towards the forehead. By bringing the head down, you make the distance to be covered much shorter, and thus the posture much easier.

If you can't lift your right foot at all, try the following simple variation of the posture. You leave the left leg stretched out, and grasp the right foot with both hands. Now it will be easier to lift the foot towards the forehead. Remember to bring the head down. Even with this simple variation you are getting most of the benefits from this posture.

The Archer Posture has many benefits. Muscles in arms, legs, shoulders and neck are all exercised, while the spine and hip joints are being loosened. Fights constipation and improves the digestive processes of the body.

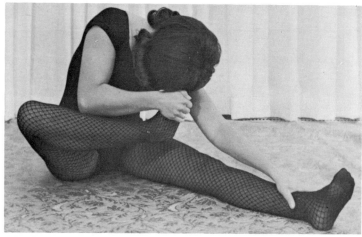

Fig. 30

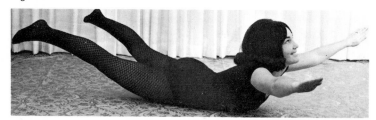

Fig. 31

Boat Posture *(Fig. 31)*

For this posture you lie flat on the floor, face down. The arms are stretched in front of the head. As you inhale deeply you raise arms, head and legs from the floor. Hold the posture as long as you can comfortably hold your breath. Should you find it too difficult to lift both arms and legs, you can try an easier variation of this posture. While you inhale deeply, raise only your arms and head from the floor. The legs stay down.

Benefits: Exercises just about every muscle in the body. Expands chest and strengthens lungs.

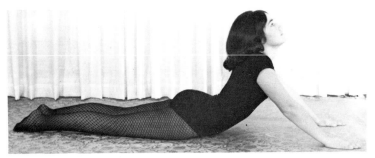

Fig. 32

Cobra Posture *(Fig. 32)*

One of the basic Yoga postures, bestowing great benefits on those who practise it. Even if your spine is not very supple, you can still perform the Cobra.

Lie on the floor, face down, keeping the feet together. Place the hands flat on the floor in front of, and outside, the shoulders. The further away you place the hands, the easier the posture becomes. As you inhale, slowly raise the head, and next the chest. So far you have not used your arms; now push yourself up further by straightening the arms, but keep the hips on the floor. Good pressure is felt in the small of the back. Hold posture for as long as you can hold your breath in comfort. Come down slowly as you breathe out.

Besides exercising the various muscles, the Cobra Posture keeps the spine elastic. Thyroid, parathyroid, adrenal and sex glands benefit greatly. An extra supply of blood is brought to the kidneys. Fights constipation and improves digestion. Highly recommended to people with backache. For women, beneficial in case of menstrual disorders, and improves the bustline.

Variation. A good bend in the back is also experienced if you rest on the elbows, which are placed directly under your shoulders. The arms can be folded. You can relax in this position; the more you relax, the more your back will bend. You can bend the legs one by one, or together, as you inhale deeply.

Camel Posture *(Fig. 33)*

Again a marvellous posture. Kneel down, with knees and feet well apart. Now lean back and try to rest the hands or fingers on your heels. As you inhale, push the abdomen forward and let your head fall back. Hold posture for as long as you can comfortably hold your breath. Should you not be able to reach your heels with your hands, try first to have your knees and feet further apart. Should you still have trouble, try to reach back with one hand only, and after a while change over and try to do the same with the other hand. Come up slowly as you breathe out.

Keeps the spine supple and strengthens the muscles along the spine, arms and shoulders. The thyroid gland is toned up, and the neck firmed. Ureter, bladder and reproductive organs benefit. The posture also helps to fight constipation and aids the digestive processes. Improves the bust. *Not to be practised by people with a hernia.*

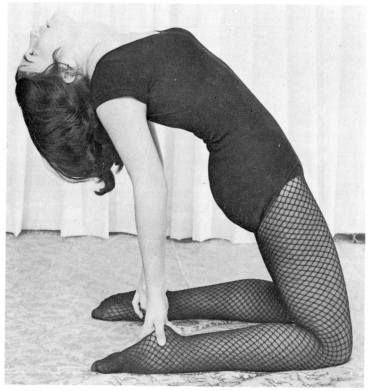

Fig. 33

Cat Posture *(Figs. 34 and 35)*

This posture is an excellent exercise for the spine along its whole length. The Cat Posture consists of two parts.

I. Get onto your hands and knees. As a cat, you are 'on all fours'. The knees are kept together, with the hands flat on the floor, well apart. Now breathe in and arch the back, bringing it up into a hump as high as you can. Your head hangs down.

40

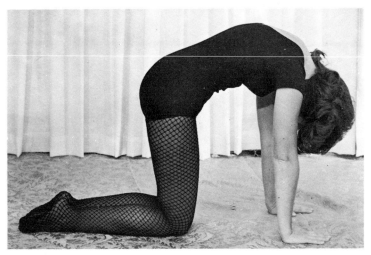

Fig. 34

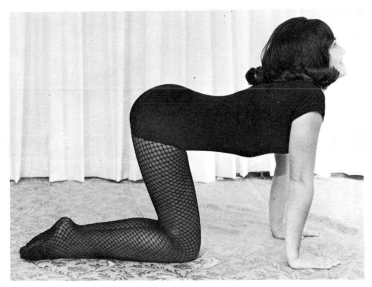

Fig. 35

II. As you breathe out, allow the body between shoulders and hips to hang down as much as possible, and bring your head up. The arms are kept straight all the time.

Beneficial for the spine, and exercises the shoulders. Women will appreciate the Cat, as it tones up the reproductive organs and helps to prevent menstrual disorders.

41

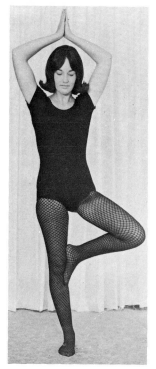 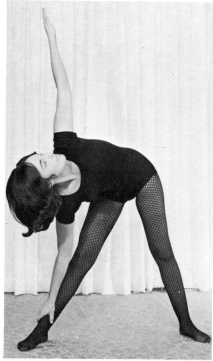

Fig. 36   *Fig. 37*

Tree Posture *(Fig. 36)*

This posture provides a simple but interesting exercise in balancing, while it strengthens feet, legs and back. First you can practise standing on the right leg.

Bring your weight onto your right leg and place the left foot against the knee. Carefully straighten up and put the hands together just above the head, with the elbows pulled back slightly to expand the chest. Hold steadily for a while. You will find it will help you to keep your balance if you stare at a point on the floor just in front of you; otherwise, gaze at a point on the opposite wall. Change legs.

Instead of placing the foot against the knee you can also lay it higher up against the thigh, with the heel near the groin.

Triangular Posture *(Fig. 37)*

Stand with the legs wide apart. As you breathe in deeply, extend the arms at shoulder height. Bend the trunk to the right as you breathe out, without turning, and with the right hand hold the right leg just above the ankle. The free arm points in the air, and you turn the head to look up as much as you can. Both legs are kept straight. Hold posture as long as is comfortable, then come up as you breathe in. Take a deep breath — you may let the arms down for a minute — then repeat posture on the other side.

Some people find the following variation of the Triangular Posture easier. Instead of bringing the right hand down the right leg, the trunk is twisted and the right hand reaches for the left ankle. You can try both methods, and practise the one you prefer.

Keeps the spine flexible and tones up spinal nerves. Abdominal region is massaged, while extra blood is brought to thyroid and parathyroid glands and the face.

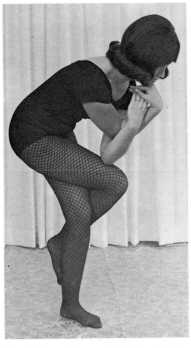

Fig. 38

Eagle Posture
(Fig. 38)

A sense of balance is acquired and further developed. Powers of concentration are improved.

Shift your weight onto your left leg, which is slightly bent. Carefully bring your right foot round the front and hook it behind the left calf. Steady yourself. Once balance has been established, twist the arms one round the other as shown in the illustration. Slowly bend forward without losing your balance and rest the elbows on the thigh. Rest the chin on the hands, and gaze at a point on the floor directly in front of you. After a while — you may hold the posture as long as you like — come back and shake the legs a little. Now balance on the opposite leg. The arms also are twisted the other way round.

The Eagle Posture strengthens feet, ankles, calves and thighs. Constipation is corrected. The sex glands are nourished and menstrual irregularities curbed. In some cases sterility is overcome.

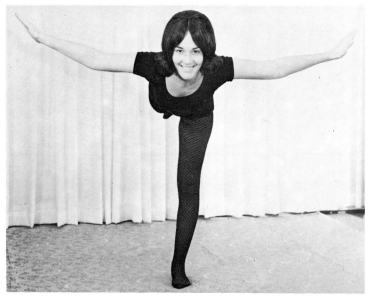

Fig. 39

Dancing Posture *(Fig. 39)*

As well as being an excellent exercise for physical balance, the Dancing Posture helps to promote steadiness of mind. Legs and muscles in the back are strengthened.

Standing first on the left leg, slowly bend forward and bring the right leg up as far as you can, keeping it straight. The arms are spread wide. You resemble a bird in flight, or an aeroplane. The final aim is to have the body horizontal, with the raised leg in line. However, in the beginning lean forward only a little. With practice you will improve.

Change legs.

Hands-to-Feet Posture *(Fig. 40)*

Stand up straight with the legs together. Bring the arms above the head while you breathe in deeply. As you exhale you lean forward and grasp the legs just above the ankles. The head is brought as close as possible to the knees. The knees must not be bent. Hold for a moment while you keep the lungs empty. Come up slowly and breathe in deeply, stretching the arms above the head.

Variation. Bend down and hold the ankles. Touch the head against the legs which are slightly bent. Keeping the forehead pressed against the knees, carefully try to straighten the legs. *It is very easy to overstrain yourself here, so be cautious.*

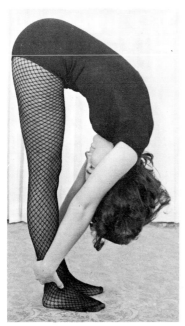

Beneficial to head, face, neck, spine, back and thigh muscles. Massages internal organs in the abdominal region, toning up liver, pancreas and kidneys. Helpful in case of menstrual irregularities, flatulence and digestive troubles.

Fig. 40

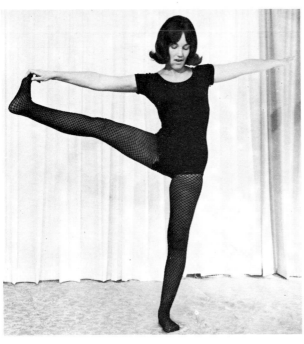

Fig. 41

One-Legged Posture *(Fig. 41)*

Posture which will help to develop a very good sense of balance, and will improve powers of concentration.

Stand up straight with the legs together. Shift your weight onto your left leg by leaning a little to the left. Slowly bring the right knee up till you can get hold of the toes with your right hand. Steady yourself first before you go any further. Carefully point the leg sideways and try to straighten the leg as much as you can. The free arm is pointing in the opposite direction and acts as a counterweight (some pretty girls can balance much better with tongue pushed into cheek!). You should not lean forward at all. Hold the posture as long as you want to, then come down and change legs.

Alternatively, you can point the leg forward instead of sideways.

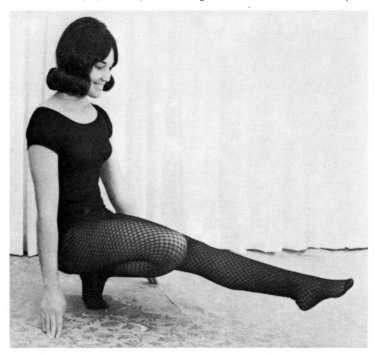

Fig. 42

Tiptoe Posture *(Fig. 42)*

Sit back on the right heel, balancing only on the toes. Support yourself on both sides with the fingers. Stretch the left leg out in front of you, keeping it horizontal and well off the floor. Once your balance in this position is established, try to bring one hand in front of the chest, still supporting yourself with the other. Finally, try to hold both hands

46

up. This is a very tricky balance. Some people may do it at their first try, while others take quite a long time to master it. No matter, it is good fun and an excellent exercise. Persevere, and you will succeed. One proud day you will sit there as steady as a statue. Change legs and try the other side.

Should you not be able to bring one leg up, just keep both legs under the body and balance that way, with the hands in front of the chest if possible.

Strengthens the feet and leg muscles. Increases flexibility of the knees. Beneficial to the pelvic area for both men and women.

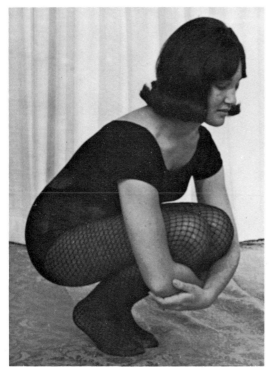

Fig. 43

Squatting Posture *(Fig. 43)*

As you come down to the squatting position, balance on the toes and support yourself with the finger-tips. Keep the feet together. Once you have a good balance, wrap the arms around the knees, drawing the knees against the body. The hands hold the elbows.

Strengthens the feet and tones up the abdominal region. Overcomes stomach upsets and menstrual disorders. Acts very powerfully against constipation.

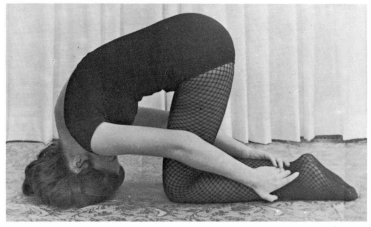

Fig. 44

Hare Posture *(Fig. 44)*

Kneel down and place the crown of the head on the floor. The buttocks are raised. The shoulders hang down, with the hands holding the legs just above the ankles. *As soon as the pressure in head and face becomes uncomfortable, the posture should be discontinued.* Come up slowly and tap face gently with the fingers.

Head and neck are supplied with fresh blood galore. Glands in the head and neck are stimulated. Facial tissues are nourished, keeping the face young and beautiful.

Half Headstand *(Fig. 45)*

True to our promise not to teach the headstand, we shall omit that well-known and most beneficial Yoga pose. In its place we have a posture which is connected with the king of Yoga postures and which in a mild way produces the same therapeutic and preventive results. It is a good substitute for the headstand, and is called the Half Headstand.

Practise on a soft yet firm surface. A folded blanket makes good padding. If you are wearing rings, make sure they don't cut into your fingers — if necessary, remove them temporarily. Kneel down and place the lower arms on your blanket. The fingers are locked, and the arms make about a sixty degree angle, so that the elbows will be directly under the shoulders. Place the head in the interlocked hands in such a way that only the hairline touches the floor. Now bring the knees off the floor and straighten the legs. You can hold this position for a moment to get used to the strange feeling, making sure your

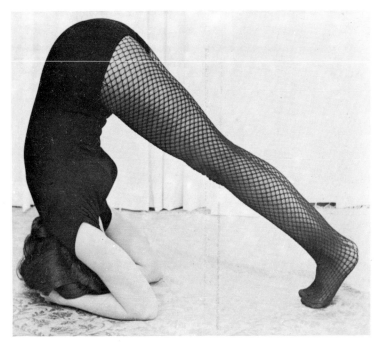

Fig. 45

fingers don't hurt. *Should the rush of blood to the head make you feel uncomfortable, come back at once, but not too suddenly.* After steadying yourself, slowly walk forward while keeping the legs straight till the trunk is in a vertical position. Keep the eyes closed. When you have held the posture long enough – that is as long as it is comfortable – drop the knees to the floor and come up slowly. Remain seated for a little while to allow the blood to flow back from the head. Pat the face gently with the fingers.

Benefits achieved by practice of the Half Headstand are manifold. The entire body is rejuvenated. The brain is nourished by an extra supply of fresh blood. Powers of concentration and memory are improved. The pituitary gland benefits, and the efficient functioning of this master gland of the body has far-reaching effects on the whole system. The facial tissues are nourished and the glands in the throat are toned up. The digestive powers are increased and constipation corrected. The ovaries are stimulated and menstrual disorders overcome. Relieves asthma and sinus complaints.

As with all inverted postures, the Half Headstand should not be practised by people with blood pressure or heart trouble. The posture should also be avoided in cases of bloodshot eyes.

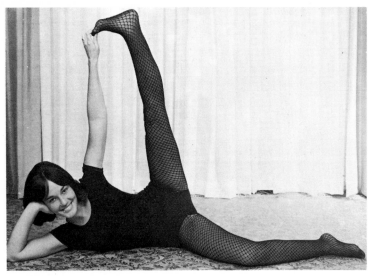

Fig. 46

One-Legged Lateral Posture *(Fig. 46)*

Instead of bringing the leg sideways when standing, here the One-Legged Posture is performed while lying down. 'Suits me fine,' some people might say.

Lie on your right side, supporting your head with the right hand. The right leg is slightly bent, which will make it easier for you to keep your balance. Get hold of the toes of your left foot with your left hand, and carefully try to straighten the leg. Hold the posture as long as you like, then bring the leg down; roll over and repeat while lying on your left side.

Strenghtens muscles at the back of the thighs and keeps the hip joints supple.

Quadruped Posture *(Fig. 47)*

How you get into this posture is a matter of discretion. You begin by lying face down with the hands placed firmly on the floor approximately under the shoulders. As you breathe in deeply, push yourself up, keeping the legs straight and the body stiff. In general, men will find the push-up much easier than women, although some girls can give a good account of themselves here. If you have trouble, you could first push the chest up, and straighten the legs afterwards. Hold breath and posture as long as is comfortable, then come down slowly as you breathe out. Rest for a moment.

The Quadruped Posture can also be practised the other way round. You sit down, with the legs in front of you, lean back and place the hands on the floor well behind you. As you breathe in, push the tips up and keep the body straight, with the head in line.

A good muscular exercise for the whole body.

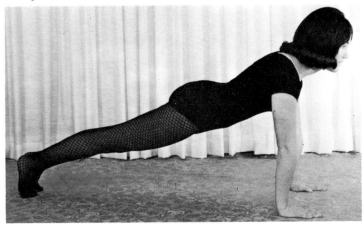

Fig. 47

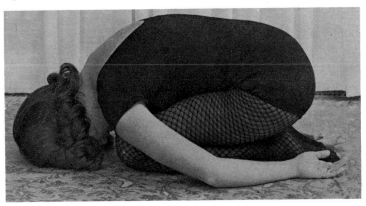

Fig. 48

Child Posture *(Fig. 48)*

Sit back on the heels as in the Thunderbolt Posture. Slowly bend forward till the forehead rests on the floor. The arms are brought back and lie limply along the body. The weight of arms and shoulders pulls on the back muscles. Breathe calmly. Should you feel the blood rush to the head too suddenly when leaning forward, try the posture in stages. Sit back on the heels, bend forward slowly and plant your elbows on the floor just in front of the knees. Now comfortably rest your chin in your hands. When you feel ready, assume the full posture.

As a variation, you could turn the head to the right instead of resting the forehead on the floor.

Besides being very restful, the Child Posture loosens the spine. Face, head and neck all receive an extra supply of arterial blood. The abdominal region is squeezed, and for this reason the Child Posture promotes good elimination.

Not to be practised by those with heart trouble or blood pressure.

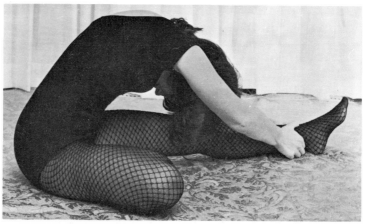

Fig. 49

Head-to-Knee Posture *(Fig. 49)*

This posture is much the same as the Posterior Stretching Posture, the difference being that only one leg is kept straight.

Sit down and fold the right leg against the body. Let the foot rest comfortably under the left thigh. Hold the left leg just above the ankle with both hands, breathe in deeply, then as you breathe out slowly pull head and trunk towards the leg. Hold for a moment while the lungs are empty, then come up as you breathe in. Change legs.

A variation for people with supple joints: instead of having the foot under the thigh, you could place the foot on top of the leg, pulling it close to the body. With this technique the pressure on the abdomen will be greatly increased.

Toe-Hold Posture *(Fig. 50)*

Lie flat on your back. Bend the legs and get hold of the toes. Try to straighten the legs slowly, but don't force things. The hips will be off the floor a little. Should you be so clever as to be able to straighten the legs completely without straining, you could try to push the hips down so that all of the back is on the floor.

Strengthens leg muscles, tones up the sciatic nerve, stimulates the ovaries and aids the digestive processes.

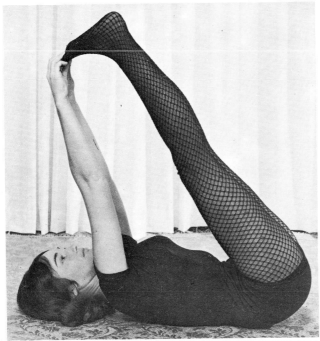

Fig. 50

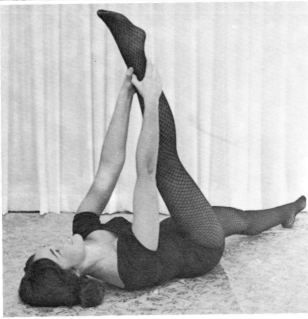

Fig. 51

53

Head-to-Leg Posture *(Fig. 51)*

Lie on your back. Slowly bend the right leg and with both hands grasp the ankle. Now try carefully to straighten the leg while the left leg remains straight and relaxed on the floor. Hold the posture and breathe calmly. Come down and change legs.

As a variation, you could try to bring the head up towards the leg, trying to touch the knee with the forehead. Keep the leg straight and the other leg on the floor.

Strengthens leg and shoulder muscles and tones up the sciatic nerve.

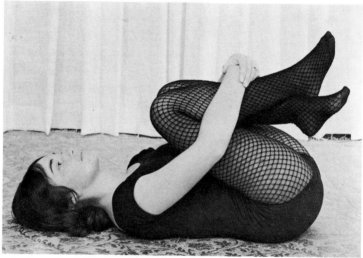

Fig. 52

Gas Ejector Posture *(Fig. 52)*

Lie on your back and draw the knees up to your stomach, with ankles crossed. Clasp the arms around the knees, pressing the knees to the body. Press only gently, and breathe slowly.

Corrects flatulence and digestive upsets. The effects of the posture can be intensified by breathing in deeply, holding the breath and pressing the knees hard to the chest. The blood will be felt rushing to the head and this extra supply of arterial blood will stimulate the facial tissues and glands in the throat. *Not to be practised in cases of hyper-tension, or by people with blood pressure or heart trouble.*

A relieving massage can be given to the back muscles by rocking gently from side to side with the knees pressed lightly to the chest. Don't rock too hard, or you'll roll over.

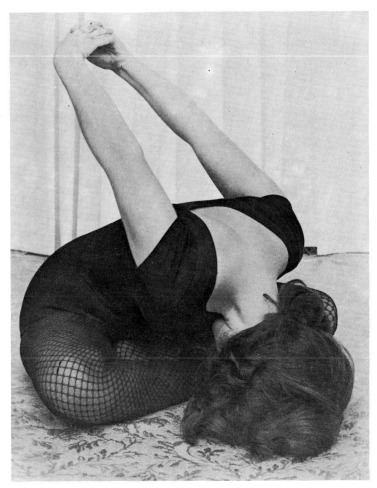

Fig. 53

Yoga Seal Posture *(Fig. 53)*

Sit with the crossed feet pulled close to the body. Make sure the ankles do not hurt on the floor. Lock the hands behind the back, and sit up while you breathe in deeply. Exhale as you slowly bend forward and bring the forehead towards the floor, at the same time raising the arms up in the air as much as you can. Hold posture for as long as you can keep the lungs empty with comfort. Come up slowly as you breathe in.

Massages abdominal region and tones up the reproductive organs. Nourishes facial tissues and glands in the throat.

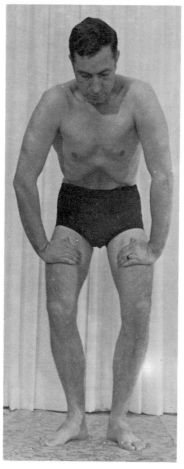

Fig. 54

Abdominal Contraction (Fig. 54)

To conclude this chapter, here is one of the most important exercises of physical Yoga. Many of the postures act to tone up the abdominal region, but this action is only mild compared to the results achieved by the properly executed Abdominal Contraction, or Uddiyana Bandha as it is called.

Stand with the feet slightly apart, and the legs bent. Lean forward, and rest the hands on the thighs. The weight of the trunk should be carried by the arms, so that the abdominal muscles are completely relaxed. Breathe in deeply, then throw the air out suddenly through the mouth. Keep the lungs empty during the exercise. Contract the abdominal muscles, drawing the stomach in and trying to bring it against the spine. Hold the contraction for as long as you can go without air, then relax the muscles and breathe in. *You should take care not to breathe in too quickly, or you may get some saliva in your windpipe.*

Try to do Uddiyana Bandha every day. It will take a while before you have fully mastered the technique and are able to make a big 'hollow' in the abdominal region. However, just the attempt is an excellent exercise. You can also try the following variation: repeatedly tense and contract the abdominal muscles in quick tempo, so that a flapping movement ensues.

Care should be taken with the Abdominal Contraction. Obviously the exercise should not be done on a full stomach. In cases of serious constipation the technique will be too severe, and should not be practised; people with ulcers should also miss it. It should not be practised during menstruation nor, needless to say, during pregnancy.

Young girls not yet fully matured would do better to forget about Uddiyana Bandha.

Go through the foregoing list of postures and familiarise yourself with them at your leisure. Learn the benefits which each posture bestows. You will find that there will be postures which will be particularly beneficial to you, and others which you will enjoy performing very much. Include all these in your programme, but make sure that the programme is well balanced. If you miss some postures at one session, try to include them the next time you do Yoga.

It would be ideal if you could practise every day. At least try to practise a few times a week. Always do some deep breathing before you start, and also some loosening-up exercises. Never hold a Yoga posture longer than is comfortable. Have sufficient rest between postures, and conclude the session with the Posture of Complete Relaxation.

You will find that you'll feel some benefits almost immediately, but that it will take a few weeks before you become appreciably more supple. From then on you will progress even more rapidly.

Go carefully, for by forcing you will not progress as you would when practising in a relaxed manner. In any case, by forcing you can do more damage than good.

4
More Exercises

Variety is the spice of life, they say, so here are some more useful exercises. You can add a few of these to your daily programme, not only for fitness and health, but also for the sake of variety.

Let us begin with some leg exercises. All these will strengthen the leg muscles considerably and really tighten up the abdominal muscles. All help to slim abdomen and waistline.

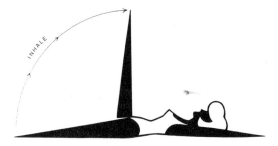

Fig. 55

1. *(Fig. 55.)* Lie on your back with the legs together and the arms stretched above the head and resting on the floor. As you breathe in, slowly raise the right leg to the vertical, keeping it straight all the while. As you breathe out, slowly lower the leg. On the following inhalation bring the left leg up, and lower it while you exhale. Now continue with the right leg and so on till you feel you have done enough.

Breathe in and out through the nose all the time, as with all these exercises.

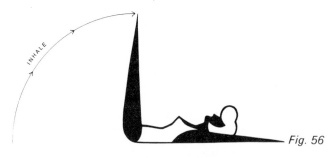

Fig. 56

2. *(Fig. 56.)* Lying on your back with arms stretched above the head, slowly raise both legs as you breathe in, till the legs are in a vertical position. As you breathe out, slowly lower the legs till they are on the

floor, always keeping the legs together. Take a slow and deep breath, then repeat the movement.

To get the most out of this exercise, you should keep the legs perfectly straight, and even have the toes in line with the legs. You will feel a marvellous pull on the abdomen as you perform this exercise.

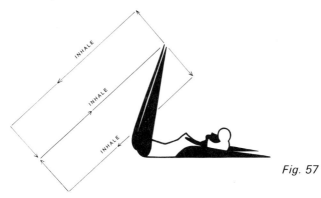

Fig. 57

3. *(Fig. 57.)* From the same supine position of the previous two exercises, bring both legs up while you breathe in. Keep legs straight and together. As you breathe out, spread the legs sideways then, keeping the legs wide apart, slowly lower them, as you breathe in, till they are just above the floor. Now bring the legs together as you breathe out. Continue in this fashion to raise, separate, lower and close the legs as often as you can without allowing them to touch the floor.

Have a little rest, then do the exercise the opposite way. Spread the legs sideways just above the floor as you breathe in deeply, slowly raise the legs as you breathe out, bring them together as you inhale, and down while you exhale.

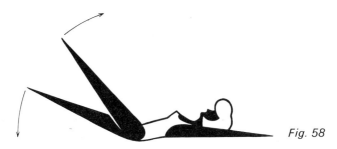

Fig. 58

4. *(Fig. 58.)* Now make some scissor movements with the legs while lying on the back. You can do this slowly and in rhythm with your breathing. Slowly raise and lower the legs one at a time without letting the feet touch the floor at all. Keep the legs straight.

59

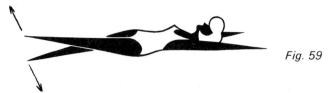

Fig. 59

5. *(Fig. 59.)* You can also make a horizontal scissor movement. First spread the legs sideways and then cross them, keeping them straight. Spread the legs again, then cross them the other way. Repeat, but stop before you get too tired.

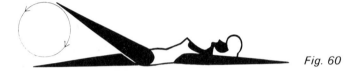

Fig. 60

6. *(Fig. 60.)* In the same position, describe a few circles with the left leg in an anti-clockwise direction. Keep the leg straight, and circle slowly. Now circle the same leg in the opposite direction.

You may have a little rest, then circle the right leg in a clockwise direction. After a few circles, move the leg the other way round. If you want to make the exercise a little harder, you can circle both legs at the same time, circling the right leg clockwise and the left anti-clockwise, then reverse the direction of both legs. Here your stomach will really feel the strain, and the legs will soon get pretty tired.

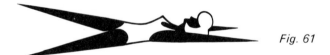

Fig. 61

7. *(Fig. 61.)* Still on your back, slowly spread the legs sideways as wide as you can while you breathe in. Keep the legs just above the floor, and slowly bring them together as you breathe out. Repeat, if you have the strength.

Fig. 62

8. *(Fig. 62.)* To make a good exercise for leg and stomach muscles, you really don't have to do much at all. Keeping the legs straight and together, just raise them half an inch above the floor and see how long you can hold them in that position unsupported.

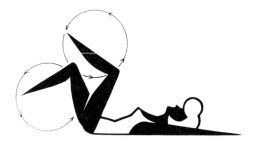

Fig. 63

9. *(Fig. 63.)* We have nearly finished the series of exercises performed while lying on the back. Raise the legs and in slow motion make cycling movements. You can cycle fast if you like. The cycling movements can also be done while the body is in the Inverted Body Posture, that is, the hips are raised and supported by the hands.

The cycling exercise has always been a great favourite with the ladies, as it helps to slim down thighs and hips.

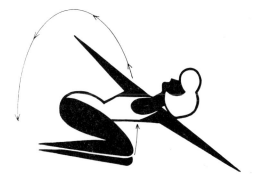

Fig. 64

10. *(Fig. 64.)* Another exercise for the hips. Lying on the back with the arms spread sideways, slowly bring the knees to the chest as you breathe in, then move them to the floor on the left of the body. Breathe out. As you breathe in, bring both knees up and over to the right. Breathe out, then bring knees over to the left again. Repeat. Breathe in every time the knees come up.

Finally, straighten the legs slowly and rest a little.

11. *(Fig. 65, page 62.)* Yet another exercise for slimming the hips, but this time you will have to sit up.

Sit on your haunches. The arms are above the head, with the hands clasped round the wrists. As you breathe in deeply, raise your hips up, cross your body over and sit down on the other side of the feet. Now slide over again, and repeat as often as you wish.

The arms stay above the head all the time. However, should you find it impossible to bring the hips up and over without help, just bring the arms down.

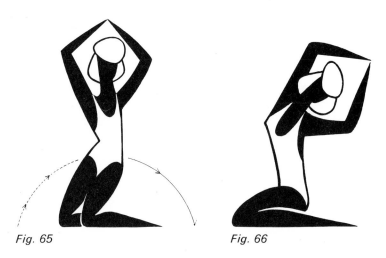

Fig. 65   Fig. 66

12. *(Fig. 66.)* To get a good pull on the muscles in the sides, you can do this sideways swing. Sit as before, with the arms above the head, breathe in deeply, and as you breathe out bounce the trunk three times to the left, without turning. Breathe in and repeat the sideways bounce. Then slide hips over the feet and bounce the trunk to the right.

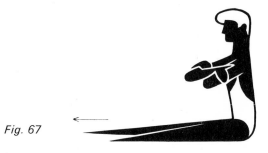

Fig. 67

13. *(Fig. 67.)* Sit with the legs stretched and together. Hold the arms shoulder high in front of you, with the hands clasped round the elbows. Now take off some weight from the hips by 'walking' on the buttocks. First thrust one leg forward as much as you can, then the other. Continue, then walk backwards.

14. *(Fig. 68.)* The rowing exercise is marvellous for the whole body. It will be hard to find a muscle which is not given a workout here.

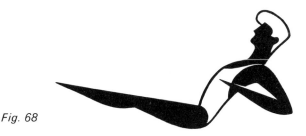

Fig. 68

Sit with the knees drawn to the chest. Reach forward with the arms and imagine you have a good grip on the oars. As you breathe in deeply, bring the feet off the floor, slowly straightening the legs as you lean backwards and pull back with the arms. As you breathe out, come back slowly to the starting position, except that the feet are kept off the floor. Remain balanced on your buttocks with knees bent. Now repeat the whole movement.

If you have had no training for rowing, and don't intend to make the national team for the Olympic Games, you can make it easier for yourself if you pause for a deep breath after each movement.

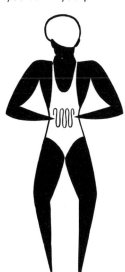

15. *(Fig. 69.)* This one is an excellent exercise for improving chest and bust as well as for strengthening arms and shoulders.

Stand with the legs somewhat apart, and hold the fists close together in front of you, with elbows pointing sideways. As you breathe in deeply, imagine you are trying to stretch a very strong spring. Don't bring the fists too far apart, say only ten inches. The spring is very strong indeed. As you breathe out, imagine you are pressing something together. Repeat several times.

Fig. 69

16. *(Fig. 70.)* Lie on your back with the hands locked behind the head. As you breathe in deeply, sit up and bounce forward with the trunk, bringing the head towards the knees. Bounce forward once more while breathing out. Lie down again as you breathe in. When you are ready, repeat the exercise.

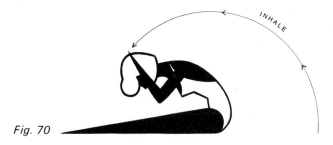

Fig. 70

Should you have trouble in sitting up, you could put your feet under, say, a low cupboard. You will find that if your feet are prevented from going up in the air, the sitting up is much easier. If you can't do the exercise at all, just practise sitting up while you are reaching forward with the arms.

Tightens up the abdominal muscles beautifully, and strengthens chest and lungs.

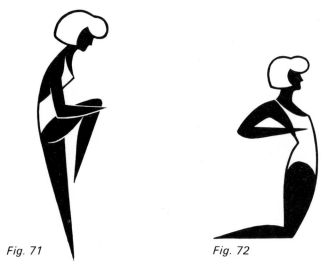

Fig. 71   *Fig. 72*

17. *(Fig. 71.)* Standing, bring the right knee up as you breathe in and, clasping hands around it, press the knee hard to the chest. Hold breath while you continue the pressure, then come down as you breathe out. Repeat with the left leg.

18. Lie face down with the arms stretched above the head. As you breathe in deeply, simultaneously bring the arms, head and legs off the floor (Fig. 31). Come down at once breathing out, and repeat several times.

An interesting variation is the following: As you inhale, bring both the right arm and the left leg up. Come down as you breathe out, then raise the left arm and the right leg as you breathe in.

19. Still lying face down, push yourself up with the arms, keeping the body straight and stiff (Fig. 57), while breathing in deeply. Holding the breath, bring one leg up, but don't move your hips. Bring the leg down again and breathe out as you slowly lower yourself to the floor. Repeat, this time bringing the other leg up.

20. *(Fig. 72.)* Resembling horse riding, this exercise will help to tighten up the thigh muscles and thus firm the thighs. Also good for chest and bust.

Sit back on the heels as in the Thunderbolt Posture (Fig. 16). Extend the arms in front of the body at shoulder height. As you breathe in, raise the body and pull back with the arms. Make sure you push the hips well forward. This will help to tone up the abdominal muscles. Sit down on the heels again as you breathe out, bringing the arms out front as before.

Continue the exercise as long as you enjoy riding the horse.

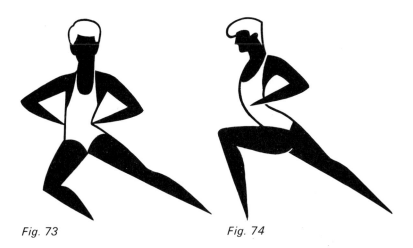

Fig. 73   *Fig. 74*

21. *(Fig. 73.)* If you want to do another exercise for leg and thigh muscles, try this. Stand with the legs very wide apart and the hands on the hips. As you breathe in, slowly bend the right leg as much as you can. Some people can go down all the way, finishing up sitting on the right heel. Come up as you breathe out, and next bend through the left leg.

22. *(Fig. 74.)* For an exercise with similar effects, imitate the movements of a fencer. Stand with the hands on the hips, slide the left foot forward as far as you can and bend the knee, while breathing in. Breathe out as you bring the legs together again, then bring the right foot forward.

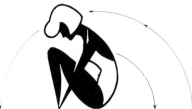

Fig. 75

23. *(Fig.75.)* Now for an exercise which will provide an excellent massage for the back muscles and the spine, and which will also tone up the nerves running along the spine. Sit on a folded blanket or a foam rubber mat. *You should not do this exercise on a very hard surface.*

Sit down and draw the legs close to the body, cross the ankles and hold the toes. Press the chin to the chest, make the back round, and let yourself fall backwards. Make sure you keep the chin to the chest, otherwise you might bang your head on the floor. Swing back and sit up again. You can do this so long as you keep your back round. Don't straighten the back while lying on the floor. As you sit up, bring the trunk forward between the knees and the forehead towards the floor. Don't swing forward too wildly, otherwise you might bounce through and hit your head on the floor. *It is better not to wear glasses here, just in case.*

24. *(Fig. 76.)* Running has always been a great conditioner, and if you get the chance, do some running or jogging out in the fresh air. You can practise in your own room by running on the spot. This can also be done in slow motion, in which case you bring the knees high up to the chest. Breathe in each time you bring a leg up, and out as you come down.

25. *(Fig. 77.)* Another exercise to send the blood rushing through your veins is this one: Stand up straight with the legs together and the arms along the sides. As you breathe in, jump the legs apart, at the same time swinging the arms up sideways and clapping the hands above the head. Jump back as you breathe out and swing arms down. Continue for as long as you think it is fun.

26. The best way to describe this exercise is to say that it is a series of Triangular Postures performed in quick succession. Stand with the legs apart and the arms out sideways, shoulder high. Breathe in

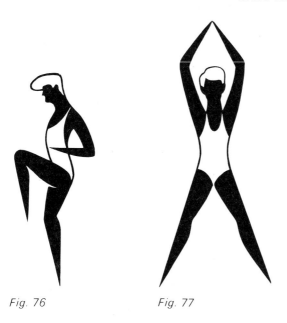

Fig. 76   Fig. 77

deeply. As you breathe out, bend forward, twist the body and with the right hand touch the left ankle (in Fig. 37 the hand touches the right ankle). The left arm points up in the air. Come up as you breathe in, and now touch the right ankle with the left hand. Repeat a few times.

27. Another quick succession of postures is our last exercise. Come down like a runner on the starting block, with the left leg bent, and the right stretched out behind you, supporting yourself on the hands. This is the same position as Step Four of the Sun Greeting (Fig. 4). Now jump and change legs, so that the right leg is bent and the left stretched out backwards, as in Step Nine of the Sun Greeting (Fig. 9). Continue, changing position in rhythm with your breathing. Should you find this exercise too easy, you could keep the legs together. First sit squatting down with the hands flat on the floor. Breathe in as you jump both legs back. You are now in the Quadruped Posture (Fig. 47). Breathe out as you jump the feet under the body again, and repeat one hundred times if you like.

5
Facts about Food and Nutrition

The human body is made up of millions upon millions of tiny living cells. All these microscopic organisms act in harmony, with each cell doing its share, enabling the body to function, to live, to work and to play. Although the cells depend on this harmonious co-operation, they are like separate and independent units, with each cell performing its function according to its own nature. For instance, the muscle cells specialise in contraction, while the speciality of nerve cells is the transmission of impulses. Each cell consists of a living membrane enclosing a semi-fluid substance called protoplasm. This protoplasm is divided into an inner core called the nucleus, and an outer portion called the cytoplasm. Fluid surrounds the cells, and from this fluid the cells take their nourishment and the required amount of oxygen. The chemical substances which nourish the cells are called nutrients.

Before it can provide nourishment for the individual cells, food has to undergo various processes. It has to be broken down physically and chemically. This happens during the journey through the digestive tract. In the mouth food is pulverised and mixed with saliva, which already exerts a chemical action upon some foodstuffs. The digestive juices produced by the body and secreted into the stomach and the small intestine mix with the food, and the various enzymes split complex food molecules into more simple molecules, while molecules of water are added. Absorption of the digested food takes place through the wall of the small intestine. Although called the 'small' intestine, the surface of this section of the digestive tract amounts to a total of about a dozen square yards. The area is so large because of the presence of many millions of finger-like processes called villi. Each villus contains a tiny blood-vessel, and so the digested material is taken up directly into the bloodstream.

Carbohydrates, fats, proteins, vitamins, minerals and water are the materials derived from food and used to promote bodily activity, growth and maintenance. Carbohydrates, fats and proteins are called 'energy foods,' because when their components are oxidized – the simpler molecules combine with oxygen – heat and energy are released. Thus the body temperature is maintained, and the cells are enabled to perform their all-important tasks. Muscles can contract, and glands produce and secrete their juices.

The liberated energy is measured in units of heat called calories. A calorie is the amount of heat needed to raise the temperature of 1 kilogram of water 1°C. On oxidation within the body, 1g. of carbohydrate and 1g. of protein each supply 4·2 calories, while 1g. of fat liberates 9·3 calories. The required daily calorie intake (in the form of carbohydrates, fats and proteins) varies greatly, depending on size, sex and body weight, and on the amount of work performed. In Western countries the energy-producing foods are readily available, and there is no shortage in the average diet; it is mostly excessive consumption leading to obesity which is the problem.

Although protein is a source of energy, its main function is the provision of material for the forming of tissues.

Vitamins and minerals assist the bodily functions, while minerals also provide material for tissue formation.

Water performs a multitude of functions, and it is present everywhere. It is the main constituent of the body, and of all the individual cells.

Carbohydrates

Starch and sugar in their various forms are carbohydrates, and we derive these mainly from plant foods. During digestion the carbohydrate compounds are broken down to simple sugars — glucose, fructose, or galactose.

Starch is the main provider of carbohydrate. It is changed during digestion to glucose. Sugars in the diet are mostly in the form of double sugars — sucrose (glucose-fructose), which is the sugar obtained from sugar beet and sugar cane, lactose (glucose-galactose), which is contained in milk, and maltose (glucose-glucose), which is found in sprouting grain. Sugars are digested rapidly, and provide therefore a more immediate source of energy than starch, the digestion of which is a longer process. Glucose is the main simple sugar derived from an ordinary diet and absorbed through the intestinal wall, while fructose and galactose occur in lesser amounts. Glucose is what we refer to when we speak of 'blood sugar.' It is transported in the bloodstream to all the cells of the tissues and organs of the body. When there is an increased supply of glucose, some of it may be stored as glycogen in different cells, especially in the cells of muscles and of the liver. Fructose and galactose are converted into glycogen in the liver and stored there as such.

The sugar level in the blood is maintained by the liver. The glycogen stored in this large organ is broken down into glucose and released into the bloodstream when the level falls below normal.

In case of over-supply, sugar is converted to fat by the liver, and stored in the fatty tissues of the body.

Fats

Fats are a concentrated source of energy. On oxidation, they provide more than twice as much energy per gram as carbohydrates and proteins. Therefore the inclusion of fats in the daily diet is of special importance when strenuous physical work has to be performed. Many fats are carriers of the fat-soluble vitamins, namely vitamins A, D, E and K. Fat can make food more palatable, while a meal containing some fat is more 'satisfying', in the sense that it takes longer to digest. Pancreatic juice and bile salts play an important role in the digestion and absorption of fats. If the fat intake is greater than the amount required for energy expenditure, the excess is stored for future use in the adipose tissues.

At room temperature, edible fats can be either solid or semi-solid 'fats', or they can be liquid 'oils'. Although both types occur in animal and vegetable sources, the solid type is more common as animal fat, such as butter and dripping, while the oils are found more in vegetable products such as olive and corn oils. Dietary fats are composed of fatty acids and glycerol. Some of these fatty acids — linoleic, linolenic and arachidonic acid — are called 'essential' because they are necessary for general good health, especially in relation to growth and healthy condition of the skin. The intake of these three essential fatty acids should be more than sufficient in any ordinary diet.

The fatty acids in the harder fats contain more hydrogen than the fatty acids of most soft fats and oils. The former are called saturated fats, and the latter are referred to as unsaturated fats. A fatty acid is 'saturated' if all its carbon atoms are fully loaded with hydrogen atoms. By a process called hydrogenation, the unsaturated fats can be converted to saturated fats. This is the case with margarine. Hydrogenation is undertaken during manufacture to make a more solid product. The measure of saturation of dietary fats has a profound influence on the level of cholesterol in the blood.

The role of cholesterol is not yet fully understood. Cholesterol is obtained from the diet and it is also synthesized in the human body. It is a waxy substance which appears in the blood and which is related to the secretions of some of the glands, while it is also involved in the transport of fat. The waxlike substance is excreted in the bile, where it is held in solution combined with bile salts. Gallstones appear if it is thrown out of solution.

Although cholesterol is regarded as essential to life, an excess of cholesterol in the blood causes fatty material to be deposited in the arterial walls, which results in their subsequent hardening, and a narrowing of those blood vessels. High blood pressure and heart disease will ensue.

Dietary cholesterol occurs in animal tissues. The principal source is egg yolk, while brains are also high in cholesterol content. Strangely, the amount of cholesterol eaten does not have an influence on the cholesterol level of the blood. This level is determined mainly by the type of fat which is consumed. Saturated fats increase, and unsaturated fats decrease, the amount of cholesterol in the blood. The unsaturated fatty acids emulsify cholesterol, thus keeping the blood vessels clear and healthy. Besides this important action, the unsaturated fatty acids fulfil another function. They nourish the nerves, and aid the formation of the myelin sheath which covers the nerves. Along with some others, the three essential fatty acids (linoleic, linolenic and arachidonic) are unsaturated.

A mixture of saturated and unsaturated fats is found in most fat-containing foods, but on the whole the unsaturated fatty acids are poorly supplied in animal fats. Fish oils are an exception. Chief vegetable sources of unsaturated fats are nuts and avocado, and the oils of wheatgerm, maize, soya bean, safflower and sunflower.

Proteins

The name 'protein' is derived from the Greek word 'proteios', which means 'holding first place'. The protoplasm of the body cells consists for a large part of protein. Muscles, nerves, organs, glands, hormones, enzymes, blood plasma, and red blood cells are all made up mainly of protein material. Nitrogen is essential for life, and protein is the only food substance which contains nitrogen. The name 'protein' is therefore aptly chosen. Without an adequate protein intake, which is needed for the renewal of the cells of the body and for the formation of new ones, there cannot be lasting good health.

During digestion, proteins are broken down to their constituent amino acids, and in the body these amino acids are synthesized to the particular proteins required by the many different and specialized tissues.

Dietary proteins differ, depending on the source from which they are derived. Foods of animal origin — milk, cheese, eggs, fish and meat — supply proteins which contain all the amino acids required, including those which cannot be synthesized in the human body from the amino acids. A total of ten amino acids cannot be synthesized in the body. These are called 'eesential amino acids', and must be supplied in the diet. The proteins derived from plant life are generally lacking in essential amino acids. Proteins which contain all the essential amino acids are called 'complete proteins' or 'first-class proteins' and those which do not contain all the essential amino acids are called 'incomplete' or 'second-class proteins'. Whole grains, soya beans, and some nuts have first-class proteins, albeit their essential amino acids are not in balanced proportions.

Proteins are also a source of energy. Where the intake of carbohydrates and fats is insufficient, the proteins of the diet — and next the proteins of the body's own tissues — are used for the production of energy, in which case there will be wastage of body tissue.

VITAMINS

Present in food in minute quantities are substances called vitamins. Their existence has been known for only a relatively short time. One of the discoverers of these all-important factors was Dr. Funk who, in 1912, isolated one form of Vitamin B which he called 'vitamine' — the final 'e' later being dropped. Since then, new vitamins have been found and their chemical identities established. Up to date, over fifteen have been discovered, and all are recognised as being essential to human life.

Vitamins are necessary for the promotion of the metabolic processes which occur within the human body. Without vitamins, various internal functions would cease and the body become diseased. Even slight deficiencies prevent maximum health and well-being. Fatigue, irritability and nervousness are some of the lesser symptoms. Where the vitamin intake is insufficient, the body's resistance to disease and infection is lowered. Serious illness can result.

Most vitamins are obtained from food, but some are produced in the intestine by bacteria.

Vitamin A is derived from carotene, a yellow pigment in many plants. It is stored in the body as a colourless compound. Vitamin A has special functions in the building of the skeleton and the teeth, and it assists the eyes in adapting to dim light. Vitamin A keeps the epithelial tissue healthy. The latter is the tissue which covers the skin and which forms the outer layer of the mucous membranes of mouth, nose, throat, eyes, inner ear, lungs, and the digestive and genitourinary tracts.

Good dietary sources of carotene are green vegetables, carrots and tomatoes. Ready-made vitamin A is found in the liver oils of sheep, halibut, cod and other oily fish. Animal fats, milk, butter and eggs are other good natural sources.

Cooking does not destroy vitamin A, but to some extent frying does.

The Vitamin B Complex. Years ago it was thought that there was just one single vitamin B, but it was soon discovered that it was really a group of different vitamins which appeared together in various foods and which worked in close relationship. The B-complex vitamins are involved in the oxidation of foodstuffs, the formation of red blood cells, and tissue activity. They help to keep skin, eyes and hair healthy. Lack of B-complex vitamins to some degree will result in listlessness, headache, nervousness, neuritis, lack of appetite, and stomach troubles.

Chief sources of the B-complex vitamins are fresh, unprocessed foods and yeast.

Thiamine (B$_1$). This important member of the group is a cure for beriberi. Thiamine is essential for good appetite, efficient digestion, and proper elimination. Along with other B-complex vitamins, it is involved in the production of the stomach's digestive juices. Thiamine is needed by the muscles of the heart and of the body. It is called the nerve vitamin, as this factor is essential for healthy nerves.

As the human body is not able to retain large quantities of thiamine, the daily diet should supply adequate amounts. Good sources are wholemeal flours and whole-grain cereals, soya beans, dried beans and peas, nuts, eggs, liver, yeast and molasses.

Thiamine is extremely soluble in water, and considerable loss occurs when cooking water is discarded. It is relatively easily destroyed by heat in alkaline media.

Riboflavin (B$_2$) is one of the vitamins which helps you to feel well and look young. It forms an important part of many enzymes found in the living cell, and plays a fundamental role in the metabolism of proteins and carbohydrates. Deficiencies are commonplace where the daily diet consists of many over-refined foods and where the intake of carbohydrates is excessive.

The eyes and the skin need riboflavin. Lack of riboflavin results in fatigue, itching and burning of the eyes, while the skin around nose and ears may become scaly. The corners of the mouth may crack, and sores on lips or face may appear.

Good sources of riboflavin are milk, liver, wholemeal cereals and flours, wheatgerm, yeast, eggs, green leafy vegetables and peas.

The riboflavin in milk is destroyed when the milk is exposed to sunlight for several hours. This vitamin of the B-complex is affected by alkalies, but it suffers little from food processing.

Niacin is the anti-pellagra factor. Together with thiamine and ribo-flavin, niacin is a constituent of the enzyme systems dealing with the oxidation of foodstuffs. Various disorders of the alimentary tract and the nervous system may be the result of a lack of niacin; digestive disturbances, nausea, diarrhoea, skin troubles, sore gums, sleeplessness, neuritis and depression can all be symptoms of niacin deficiency.

Excellent sources of this vitamin are organ and muscle meats such as liver, kidney and heart, wholemeal flours and cereals, wheatgerm, yeast and green leafy vegetables.

Cyanocobalamin (B$_{12}$). This vitamin with the long name was discovered in 1948, and was found to be essential for the formation of red blood cells. It is a very potent factor, and is best known as a cure for pernicious anaemia. Cobalt is an essential part of the vitamin B$_{12}$ molecule.

Cyanocobalamin plays a role in the growth of children, and it is needed for full physical vigour, mental alertness and the adaption to stress. Migraine, trigeminal neuralgia, oedema, osteo-arthritis, glossitis and liver ailments can all result from a shortage of vitamin B_{12}.

Chief sources of vitamin B_{12} are organ and glandular meats, eggs and fish. Milk also contains some of this vitamin.

Folic Acid is also essential to the formation of red blood corpuscles, and is therefore another anti-anaemia vitamin. Symptoms of deficiency can be various gastro-intestinal disorders, and an inadequate amount of stomach acid. When folic acid is in good supply, it helps to increase the appetite and brings about a general feeling of wellbeing.

The important sources of folic acid are organ and glandular meats, and yeast. Some of the vitamin occurs in green leafy vegetables and several other foods.

Pantothenic Acid influences the metabolism of carbohydrates, and promotes healthy adrenal glands and favourably affects the nervous system. Healthy hair and smooth facial skin are two of the results of a sufficient pantothenic acid intake.

Sources of this vitamin are liver, kidney, heart, eggs, molasses, peas and peanuts.

Choline is a fat-dissolving agent. It helps to prevent fatty degeneration of the liver, and is concerned with the distribution of fat in the right places throughout the body. The human body needs this member of the vitamin B- complex for the utilisation of cholesterol. The next two members of this group — inositol and pyridoxine — work closely together with choline in preventing cholesterol from settling in the arteries, and are thus important factors in the fight against the hardening of the arteries. Choline is also concerned with the transmission of nerve impulses.

Dietary sources of choline are meats — especially organ meats — eggs, milk, green vegetables, and wholemeal flours and cereals.

Inositol helps choline to protect the liver, and assists with the distribution of fat. Inositol is also involved in the regulation of peristalsis of the intestine. The muscles need inositol, in particular the heart muscles.

Dietary sources are meats, liver, kidney, heart, brain, soya beans and citrus fruits.

Pyridoxine (B_6). The nervous system depends on pyridoxine for good health. This vitamin is involved in the metabolism of proteins, and it is an anti-infection factor. Deficiency may result in digestive and intestinal disorders, nausea, neuro-muscular ailments, skin disorders and insomnia.

Chief sources of pyridoxine are liver, wholemeal flours and cereals, wheatgerm, yeast and molasses.

Vitamin C, also referred to as ascorbic acid, is essential for the proper formation and the health of the connective tissue in which all the cells of the body are embedded. Invading bacteria and viruses are offered strong resistance if the connective tissue is in a healthy condition. Vitamin C is also involved in the formation of the red blood cells. Children need vitamin C for healthy growth of their bones. A sufficient intake of vitamin C is necessary for general health; it helps to strengthen the walls of the blood vessels, and also strengthens sinews and ligaments. With an inadequate intake of vitamin C, the teeth may become decayed, the gums become soft and spongy, and bleed and the teeth fall out. The bones do not calcify properly and bone disease may occur. They break easily and mend slowly. The joints become swollen and tender, and later immovable. The skin bruises quickly, and wounds heal with difficulty. In cases of severe deficiency, damage to the heart muscles may occur.

In the old days, when the sailing ships made far journeys and were at sea for a long time, scurvy wrought havoc among the ship crews. Officers of the British Navy discovered – this was about 200 years ago – that lime juice prevented this dreaded disease. Ever since, citrus fruits have been used as a prevention of scurvy.

Oranges, grapefruits and lemons are the best sources of vitamin C, but the vitamin also occurs pentifully in many other fresh fruits and vegetables.

Cooking, preparation and storage all result in much loss.

Vitamin D assists in the absorption of calcium and phosphorus from the small intestine, and plays an important role in the calcification of the bones. It is thus essential for the formation of strong bones and teeth. Children who suffer from lack of vitamin D develop rickets. In adults, the bones become porous.

Vitamin D has various other important functions. It is, for instance, involved in the clotting of blood, and aids normal action of the heart.

Oily fish are a good source of vitamin D, while the vitamin also occurs in certain foods of animal origin, such as eggs and milk.

Vitamin D is formed in the human body through the action of ultra-violet light on the skin. The oil glands of the skin secrete a provitamin, and through the action of the ultra-violet rays of the sun this provitamin is converted into vitamin D, which the body absorbs through the skin.

Cooking, preservation and storage have little effect on food's vitamin D content.

Vitamin E is widely spread throughout the body, and affects many varied processes. Its full significance is not yet completely appreciated. Vitamin E is involved with fat metabolism, and it is essential for the proper functioning of the endocrine glands. The heart and the blood vessels need vitamin E, while it also helps to prevent the formation of blood clots. The oxygen requirement of the muscles is decreased sharply by the presence of vitamin E.

Vitamin E is thought to have an influence on the reproductive capacity of both sexes. It has been suggested that in some cases sterility was due to a lack of this vitamin. Vitamin E is widely distributed in foods, so there is little likelihood of deficiency in a wholesome diet. Wheatgerm is a rich source of vitamin E, while it is also present in green leafy vegetables and, in small amounts, in various other foods.

Vitamin K plays an important role in the clotting of blood, thus preventing haemorrhages. It is found in many foods, and especially in green vegetables. Adequate amounts should be obtained from the average diet, while the human body produces more of the vitamin by bacterial synthesis in the intestines.

Vitamin P is essential for strong and healthy capillaries. Vitamin P, which is really a complex, works in close association with vitamin C, enhancing the effectiveness of the latter. These two vitamins, so closely allied in function, appear together in their natural state. Fruits, especially citrus fruits, and vegetables are the chief dietary sources.

MINERALS

Minerals form an essential part of the body's skeleton, tissues and fluids. They play a vitally important role in the regulation of the body's various functions. For example, minerals are involved in the contraction of muscles and the beat of the heart, they are needed for the utilisation of nutrients, they control the water balance in the body, and they are necessary for a healthy nervous system. Most ordinary mixed diets supply sufficient amounts of the minerals required by the human body, but there could be a shortage of calcium and iron. In some areas, the iodine content of locally grown food may be very low.

Calcium is the mineral which occurs in the greatest amount in the body. It builds the bones and renders them strong, and makes the teeth hard and resistant to decay. Calcium is an essential constituent of the bodily tissues, the digestive juices and the blood plasma. Calcium plays a role in the clotting of blood, is essential for the swift transportation of nervous stimuli, and is needed for the proper utilisation of iron. Calcium promotes the health and efficiency of the muscles. The heart depends on calcium for its constantly repeated contraction. Some of the minor signs of calcium deficiency in the diet may be irritability, nervous tension and muscle cramps.

As calcium is being used all the time, the body's supply must be regularly replenished in the diet. A generous daily supply will not only guard against deficiency, but will make a real contribution to health and well-being. Although adults no longer need calcium for the formation and growth of their bones and teeth, a sufficient supply is essential if the bones are to remain strong. In case of gross deficiency the blood calcium level falls significantly, the bones give off calcium to the blood.

Milk and cheese are especially rich in calcium. Other dietary sources are molasses, lemons, oranges, eggs, oatmeal, turnips, spinach and asparagus.

Phosphorus is an essential constituent of each cell nucleus. It is next in quantity in the body to calcium, and works in close association with the latter mineral. Some of the absorbed phosphorus cannot be utilised if insufficient calcium is consumed. Phosphorus combines with calcium to make strong bones and teeth, and it fulfils various other functions. It assists in the absorption of fats and sugars, and aids in the process of converting these nutrients into energy.

Foods of animal origin generally contain more phosphorus than do vegetables and fruits.

Iron is most important for the absorption of oxygen from the air in the lungs, and for the subsequent oxidation of food nutrients in the cells — vital functions indeed. It is a component of the red colouring matter of the red blood corpuscles which is called haemoglobin. Because iron has a physical attraction for oxygen, it takes up oxygen as it passes through the capillaries of the lungs. In the bloodstream the iron-oxygen combination (called oxyhaemoglobin) is transported to the cells.

Although the red blood corpuscles have a relatively short life, the human body conserves the iron contained in those worn-out cells. Therefore only very little iron has to be supplied in the diet, unless injury or haemorrhages occur. Because of their periodic loss of blood, women do need additional supplies of iron.

The body only absorbs iron from food when needed. A shortage of iron results in excessive tiredness, low blood pressure and nutritional anaemia.

Excellent sources of iron are eggs, liver, heart, kidney, fish, yeast and whole wheat. Green leafy vegetables and dried fruits such as prunes, raisins and apricots are also good dietary sources of iron.

Iodine is present in the body only in small amounts, but it is an essential mineral all the same. Iodine is a constituent of the hormone secreted by the thyroid gland, and thus it is intimately involved in the regulation of the body's functions. Iodine deficiency results in disorder of the thyroid gland, causing it to enlarge and develop goitre. The metabolism of the body is slowed down.

All saltwater fish and other seafoods are excellent sources of iodine. Seaweeds are especially rich in iodine, and they provide an industrial source of the mineral. Iodine also occurs in vegetables. In some inland areas the soil and the water lack iodine, and there goitre is a common disease.

Potassium helps to keep the nervous system healthy. It is essential for a strong and regular heartbeat.

Magnesium is important in regard to the relaxation of the body's muscles.

Fluorine is present mainly in the teeth and the bones. The principal source of this mineral is water, while it also occurs in various foods.

Sodium, chlorine, sulphur, manganese, bromine, copper, cobalt and zinc are the other minerals present in the human body. Deficiency of these is most unlikely with any normal diet.

WATER

Water makes up about two-thirds of a human being's weight. It is involved in all the functions of the body, while it also regulates the loss of heat, thus controlling the temperature of the body. Man can do without food for weeks on end, but he can live without water for perhaps only a few days.

Loss of water occurs in the excretion of urine and faeces, and by evaporation from the lungs and the skin. Average daily requirement for an adult living in a moderate climate is approximately $4\frac{1}{2}$ pints. In case of excessive perspiration this amount would be much greater. Here there is considerable salt loss, and this should be replaced.

Food consists for a great part of water, while within the body water is produced by the metabolism of carbohydrates, fats and proteins. This accounts for about half the daily need, and the remainder must be obtained from the drinking of fluids. When more water is drunk than needed, the kidneys excrete the surplus, while the amount of water in the blood and in the tissue will remain at normal levels.

Although it would certainly be a fascinating study, there is no need for the average person to graduate in biochemistry. Some knowledge of the basic principles of sound nutrition, however, will prove to be worthwhile knowledge indeed. Of course, to be of any use, this knowledge will have to be brought into practice in daily life. You cannot expect your body to perform perfectly, and you cannot hope to feel and look your best, if you don't eat properly.

6
Eating for Youth and Health

Eating habits are usually acquired in childhood and continued throughout life. Not always are these habits correct. Diets often include too many foodstuffs of the wrong kind, and not enough of the essential nutrients. No allowance is made for the changing demands of the body. In middle age people continue to devour the enormous meals they used to eat during adolescence. Such incorrect eating habits over a prolonged period give rise to serious complaints, especially later in life. Overeating causes much more trouble than just an oversized waistline. Diabetes, arteriosclerosis, high blood pressure, and heart trouble are self-inflicted maladies in most cases.

Even in countries where food is plentiful and cheap, not all people are well fed, albeit they get enough to eat. Frequently the calcium intake is insufficient, while all too often there is a glaring lack of vitamins in the daily diet. Eating well really means much more than loading the stomach to its full capacity at every dinner session. Although the stomach may be filled, some of the bodily tissues might not receive the specialised nourishment they crave. Deficiency in vital nutrients is the underlying cause of many diseases.

The health-conscious person selects his food with care, ensuring that every single item he chooses contributes something to his physical well-being. He will eat foods which are rich in proteins, vitamins and minerals. Eating those foods means promoting health, vigour, good looks and longevity. It means protection against disease and premature old age. The human body cannot remain in first-class order if it is supplied with inferior materials. High-starch foods such as white bread, cakes, pies and sweets do little more for the body than appease the appetite and put on weight. They slow down and interrupt the digestion of the more wholesome foods, and restrict the intake of those superior foodstuffs.

If you want to be as healthy as possible — and it will be difficult to think of many better investments — you will have to watch what you eat. Make sure that your body receives all the nutritive elements it needs. Get plenty of first-class proteins, and eat fresh fruits and vegetables in abundance. You must learn fully to appreciate nature's own foods. Man cannot copy the exquisite flavours brought out by nature. How can he imitate the goodness and taste of a fresh baby carrot, a sun-kissed orange, or golden honey gathered by the bees from many beautiful flowers?

Protein Foods

No matter what age you are, it is of paramount importance that your protein intake is adequate. Health, strength and vitality are dependent on the tissue-building proteins. Without them, the body goes soft and flabby, and becomes susceptible to infection.

Most nutritionists agree that under normal circumstances a man's daily diet should contain about 100 grams of proteins, with the requirements for women being slightly less. At least half of this should be made up of the first-class proteins derived from animal sources. A vegetarian diet is more likely to be satisfactory if it includes milk, cheese and eggs.

All meats are excellent sources of good-quality proteins, while the glandular meats, such as liver, kidney and heart, are rich also in vitamins and minerals. Fish is comparable with meat in composition. It contains first-class protein and B-complex vitamins, especially nicotinic acid. The iron content of fish is lower than that of meat, but on the other hand, fish contains much more iodine. In addition, the oily fish are an excellent source of vitamins A and D, while the edible bones make a considerable contribution to the calcium intake.

Eggs, designed by nature to nourish the young chicken, have a high nutritive value. They are a rich source of first-class protein, iron and vitamin A. Eggs also supply fat, calcium, phosphorus, thiamine, riboflavin and vitamin D. All these valuable elements are contained in the yolk, while the white consists almost entirely of protein. It makes no difference whether eggs are eaten alone or as a constituent of other dishes. No advantage is gained by eating eggs raw; actually, they are more easily digested when eaten lightly cooked.

Following are the protein contents of some popular foods:

1 pint of milk	17g. of protein
½ cup of powdered skim milk	21g. ,,
½ cup of wheatgerm	4g. ,,
½ cup of fresh peas	5g. ,,
½ cup of dried peas	7g. ,,
1 serving of breakfast cereal	2g. ,,
1 serving of vegetables	1g. ,,
1 serving of meat, fish or poultry	18g. ,,
1 serving of fruit	1g. ,,
1 slice of bread	2g. ,,
1 medium egg	6g. ,,
1 medium potato	3g. ,,

The human body has two digestive systems — an alkaline system for the digestion of carbohydrates, and an acid process for the digestion of proteins. The carbohydrates are acted upon by the saliva, which has an alkaline base. Further digestion of carbohydrates takes place in the upper part of the small intestine. Carbohydrate foods should be chewed well, but this does not necessarily hold true for protein foods. The digestion of proteins takes place principally in the stomach by the gastric juices which have as their main constituent hydrochloric acid. The latter is a very strong acid which does an effective job in breaking down protein foods, while it also is a powerful germ killer. Nature provides us with a look at two different digestive systems in action. The herbivorous cow chews long and patiently, while the carnivorous lion tears off large chunks of meat and swallows them whole. Yet the lion can jump much further than the cow (this would also make a good case for the consumption of first-class protein foods!). Anyway, the stomach juices do a very thorough job in digesting protein foods, with mastication having little effect. It has even been suggested lately that too much chewing makes the digestion of protein foods more difficult.

Fruits and Vegetables

Fresh fruits and vegetables abound with vitamins and minerals, and therefore you should daily eat a wide variety of these healthy foods. Remember the old saying: 'An apple a day . . .' Of course, fruit is on its own as far as flavours are concerned.

In order to get the full vitamin value, you should eat fruits and vegetables while they are still fresh. These foods lose their vitamin C fairly quickly, especially if they are bruised or torn during picking, packing or transport. Further loss occurs during storage, particularly if they are not stored in an adequately cooled place. It is therefore false economy to buy wilted vegetables or damaged fruits.

Not only should vegetables be bought wisely, but they should also be prepared with knowledge and care. Shredding, grating and chopping all result in vitamin C loss, as this vitamin is oxidized by the oxygen in the air. The knife used should be sharp, and the vegetables should be prepared at the last moment. Washing under running water is preferable to soaking. Where possible, peeling should be avoided. Vegetables should be short-cooked, in a minimum amount of water, and served as quickly as possible. The cooking water should not be discarded, as it will contain water-soluble minerals plus vitamins B, C and P. This water can be used, for instance, for soup. In case of over-cooking, the water may become more valuable than the vegetables!

The indigestible part of vegetables and grain products is cellulose, but even this plays its role, as it provides the bulk necessary for the peristalic contractions of the bowels.

Canned and frozen vegetables are usually good value for money if no fresh varieties are available. Dehydrated vegetables may be low in vitamin C, unless modern drying methods have been used.

As all fruits are carbohydrates, their digestion begins in the mouth.

Nature intended fruits to be eaten, as saliva is a digestive juice. During mastication, the saliva is thoroughly mixed with the fruit, and thus the first stage of the digestive process can take place. Fruit juice, when taken in quantity, may not be completely digested, and may even upset various chemical processes within the body. Therefore, fruit juice should be sipped slowly, and not taken in large amounts at the one time.

Fruits and vegetables aid in maintaining the alkaline condition of the blood. Grapefruit, oranges and lemons do not produce an acid reaction. This may seem strange, but the reason is that they form different combinations during digestion. The acid fruits actually help to reduce acidity.

Potatoes

Potatoes are a starchy vegetable, but a good food all the same. They contain vitamins A, B-complex and C, plus several important minerals and a small amount of protein. Their vitamin C content decreases during storage, but new potatoes steamed in their jackets are an excellent source of ascorbic acid.

In many parts of the world, potatoes are underrated as a nutriment. This is not the case in Holland, where they form a substantial part of every main dish. And the Dutch build mighty dikes! The author remembers well how during World War II in the big cities in Holland people knocked on doors to ask the occupants for only one single potato. A tale of misery and great hunger usually made the occupants surrender a potato from their own meagre rations. However, it was soon discovered that the door-knockers worked at this job full-time. A little arithmetic showed that the beggars accumulated a great hoard of the treasured food items during an honest(?) day's work, and that their activities brought them a small fortune on the black market. An interesting example of free enterprise in occupied territory!

Milk

Milk is a most excellent food, which is understandable seeing that nature intended it to be the sole sustenance of the newly-born. Milk is easily digestible and contains most of the essential food elements. It is a rich source of protein, calcium and phosphorus, and it contains the whole range of known vitamins. The protein in milk is first-class protein, and thus equally as good as the protein in meat and eggs. The fat in milk is finely emulsified, and therefore readily digested. Many diets are deficient in first-class proteins, calcium and riboflavin, with the result that people get old physically before their time. By adding one pint of milk to their daily diet, these people will be able to enjoy the prime of life much longer. Milk helps to keep you young and healthy.

While milk is almost the perfect food, it is deficient in iron. The amounts of vitamins C and D it contains are also not very high.

Underweight can be caused by disease and glandular disorder, but in many cases underweight people can build themselves up by doing plenty of exercises, by eating plenty of good foods, and by drinking plenty of milk.

A glass of milk usually helps to relieve acidity and indigestion, as it has an alkaline reaction in the stomach. For this reason older people, whose digestive acid may have lost some of its strength, would be wiser not to drink too much milk with meals. It may interfere with their stomach's digestion of proteins and iron-containing foods. Older people should drink milk, but they should drink it between meals. It can be taken in any form or in any beverage.

The pasteurisation of milk does not lower its nutritive value, but the process does further lower the milk's vitamin C content, while there is also some loss of thiamine. The same holds true for the condensation of milk.

Powdered skim milk contains all the important nutritive elements of fresh milk, with the exception of fat and the fat-soluble vitamins. The latter are, however, amply supplied in the average diet. Powdered skim milk is a wonderful concentrated food which can be put to many good uses. It is high on proteins and low on calories, and can be applied as a fortifier of many dishes and drinks. Try scrambled eggs mixed with powdered skim milk for breakfast!

Cheese contains all the valuable protein, minerals and vitamins of milk. An ounce of cheese is approximately equal in protein content to an ounce of meat or one medium egg. Cheese can be blended beautifully with the constituents of many varied dishes.

Yoghurt

Yoghurt is a healthy, palatable and easily digested food. It contains many of the best properties of milk.

Yoghurt is made by seeding warm milk with the culture Lactobacillus Bulgaricus (which evidently shows that yoghurt was invented in Bulgaria, home of many centenarians). The culture converts the milk sugar into lactic acid, which causes the milk to thicken.

The bacteria in yoghurt fortify the stomach acid and aid in the body's absorption of vitamins and calcium as well as other minerals. They kill harmful bacteria in the colon, and promote the elimination of waste products.

Yoghurt is delightful when eaten on its own, or with the addition of honey, molasses, brown sugar, or various fruits.

Wholemeal Bread

Wheat and other cereals have a high carbohydrate content (approx. 70%) and are therefore good energy foods. They also contain a substantial proportion of protein (approx. 11%), iron and phosphorus, while they are excellent sources of B-complex vitamins. Sadly, though, the bread you buy at your local baker does not always supply you with all this goodness.

Wheat is converted into flour by milling. In order to improve the colour of the flour, the wheatgerm and the bran are removed. The result is a beautifully white product (robbed of most of its valuable nutrients). The mill offal is used for poultry and stock feed. The animals don't mind the colour, for they thrive on the offal. Small wonder, for the wheatgerm and the bran between them contain by far most of the valuable parts of the wheat.

In 100% wholemeal bread, all of the flour is used, and thus all of the goodness of wheat reaches you. During baking, however, some loss of thiamine occurs. Toasting of bread causes further loss of this vitamin.

In order to improve the quality of white bread, the sifted flour is artificially fortified in most countries.

Wheatgerm

The germ of the wheat is really an embryo, like the yolk of an egg, and it contains the nutrients for the new plant. Like egg yolk, wheatgerm is an excellent concentrated food. The oil of wheatgerm is a rich source of vitamin E, a factor not found in great amounts in other foods. Wheatgerm richly supplies thiamine, often labelled the nerve vitamin. Wheatgerm further contains many other B-complex vitamins, protein and minerals, especially phosphorus, calcium and iron.

A most nourishing breakfast food can be made by pouring hot or cold milk over wheatgerm, and adding some honey and pieces of fruit. As a natural fortifier, wheatgerm can be sprinkled over many foods. It is now readily available from any Health Food store. As the product is highly perishable, it should be kept under refrigeration.

Molasses

As is the case with wheat, nutritional sacrifices have been made for the sake of visual appeal in the manufacture of white sugar. The sugar cane is rich in vitamins and minerals, but after milling and refining the resulting white sugar is completely devitamised and demineralised. The product looks beautiful perhaps, but it is nothing but 100% starch, supplying the user only with sweetened calories. The goodness remains in the molasses, which is the residue. Molasses is mixed with cattle food and, as is the case with wheatgerm and bran, it is highly appreciated by the animals.

Molasses is rich in potassium and calcium, while it contains relatively large amounts of phosphorus and iron. Even a little copper is found in molasses. Copper is involved in the conversion of dietary iron into haemoglobin. Molasses also contains various B-complex vitamins, with inositol being especially well represented.

Unsulphured molasses is available for human consumption, and can be used as a sweetener in many ways.

Honey

The principal constituent of honey is dextrose. This is the sugar to which all carbohydrates must be broken down before they can be converted into glycogen, the body sugar. Honey is therefore a pre-digested sugar, and a ready source of energy. Not only is honey nature's own exquisite sweetening agent, but it also contains valuable food elements. Vitamin C is present in honey, and this vitamin is retained longer than in most vegetables and fruits. Honey also contains several of the B-complex vitamins, along with some minerals, hormones and a small amount of protein. Honey is a protective food, as it is a powerful germ killer. It is also a mild laxative. Altogether, honey has much more to contribute to health than does bleached white sugar. Honey should therefore be on the table of every health-conscious person.

The Enemies of Vitamins

Drugs are the enemies of vitamins, for they hinder the absorption and beneficial effect of these most important factors. The taking of drugs, therefore, should be discontinued as soon as permission is obtained from the physician. Aspirin interferes especially with the actions of vitamins C and D, while thiamine is destroyed by the barbiturates which are widely used as sedatives.

Paraffin oil laxatives coat the intestines and thus prevent the absorption of the fat-soluble vitamins A, D, E and K. Smoking destroys a considerable amount of vitamin C, and alcohol is the enemy of the vitamins of the B-complex.

Tea and coffee contain the drug caffeine, which is a mild stimulant. Taken in moderation, these beverages cause little harm. Tea and coffee in themselves have no food value, but the added sugar (brown!) and milk have. When coffee is made solely with milk it becomes a nutritious drink.

In general, it is better to eat the foods which are rich in vitamins than to take synthetic preparations of vitamins to supplement the diet. Foods contain more than vitamins. However, should there be any doubt about the vitamin content of the available food, then vitamin pills can be of great help.

Excitement, worry, anger or irritation all disrupt the process of digestion. Meals should be eaten unhurriedly, in a peaceful mood, and with joy; this will actually aid digestion. Lack of appetite can have many causes, but it is often brought on by mental strain. It could also be caused by lack of thiamine in the diet.

Overloading the stomach is a common cause of indigestion; therefore you should always stay well within the stomach's capacity. Enough is as good as a feast. The digestion of a heavy meal calls on all the resources of the system, and this will leave you without energy required to fulfil your tasks. And eating a heavy meal just before retiring at night will not give you a restful sleep. The last meal of the day should be taken early in the evening.

Breakfast should be a nourishing meal. Tea and toast may temporarily satisfy the appetite, but it certainly does not present adequate nourishment. The body has been without food for about twelve hours, and fresh nutriment is required. Instead of being only white-bread toast, your first meal of the day should contain plenty of protein, vitamins and minerals. This way you will feel better, your nerves will be steadier, you will be able to think more clearly, and you will work more efficiently. Skipping breakfast altogether may lead to 'that tired feeling' halfway through the morning. Those who take only a cup of black coffee before they rush off to work do themselves a grave injustice. They are taking a stimulant while denying themselves the corresponding nourishment.

Eating regularly at set intervals will discourage the eating of those in-between-meals snacks for which there is no need. Instead of drinking countless cups of tea or coffee during the day, you would be wiser to drink milk, fruit juice, or just plain water.

7
Reducing the Sensible Way

There are more disadvantages to being grossly overweight than the mere aesthetic aspect. Life insurance companies set much higher premiums for obese people than for persons of normal weight. And small wonder, for obesity is a serious health hazard. Excessive weight means an extra burden not just on the legs, but on heart, lungs, and digestive organs. The likelihood of the occurrence of circulatory disorders, diabetes, liver complaints, kidney and gall-bladder trouble, arthritis and gout is much greater in the obese. Being fat is also a handicap should surgery be called for, while for women the risk of complications in pregnancy increases.

Added strain is put on the heart of the overweight person. The surrounding fat restricts the heart's pumping action, while at the same time more blood has to be pumped to all the adipose tissues. Most overweight persons overeat on starches, fats and sugars. The heavy consumption of animal fat and starches causes cholesterol to deposit in the arteries, which increases the risk of coronary attack enormously. Some people tolerate a high cholesterol level in the blood, while in others it results in heart failure at a much-too-early age.

New sensational diets appear regularly in the daily papers and in the weekly magazines. Nearly all of these slimming regimes depend on a drastic reduction of the calorie intake, with some being more effective than others. On the whole, however, these crash diets have little lasting effect. The initial enthusiasm of the reducer soon wanes, and he reverts to his old habits. Who wants to live on nothing but eight eggs a day for the rest of his life, or exist solely on milk and bananas?

Some advertised diets are sub-standard, and leave the reducer in an under-nourished state, prone to infection and disease. He becomes tired, nervous and irritable, and tries to ease his troubles with alcohol, tobacco or drugs. Some slimming gimmicks are outright dangerous, and result in an aftermath of serious disorders.

In any diet it is important that the nutritional requirements of the body are met. The reducer must restrict his intake of carbohydrates and fats, but sufficient protein, minerals and vitamins should be eaten. Minerals and vitamins don't put on weight, and protein of course is essential for good health. It is not much fun being slim but sick.

Various drugs are used in the fight against obesity, but drugs should be taken only in extreme cases, and under strict medical supervision.

Indiscriminate use of drugs can have serious side-effects. The sensible person will exercise his will-power rather than rely on dangerous drugs. It is only in very few people that obesity is caused by endocrine disturbance.

The human appetite mechanism is not yet fully understood, but psychological factors are involved. Until recently it was held that the appetite was regulated by contractions of the stomach. Now, however, it is known that the appetite is governed from centres at the base of the brain. Habits play a role, as do the appearance, smell, and taste of food. The mind can be re-educated, and the appetite controlled.

There is no magic formula for losing weight other than being physically more active and eating less of the high-calorie foods. The expenditure of energy expressed in calories must be higher than the intake of calories. The secret of slimming is as simple as that. Eat fewer calories than you expend. Losing weight without showing some restraint at the dinner table is a near-impossibility.

Energy is being used up all the time. Even when you are doing nothing, the heart continues to beat, the breathing action goes on, and various bodily functions take place. The energy expended when a person is at complete rest — physically and mentally — eighteen hours after the last meal, is called the 'basal metabolic rate'. It is proportional to the surface area of the body. The basal metabolic rate for the average man is about 75 calories per hour, and for the average woman approximately 65 calories per hour. So even while you are asleep, you burn up the calories — a comforting thought for reducers.

The daily energy requirements vary too much for different people to be stated as an exact figure. The main determinant is the amount of physical activity, but other factors also play important roles. We can only say that the average man of medium height and medium build, doing an average amount of work in a moderately active job during a normal day, expends approximately 3000 calories. Similarly, the average housewife who does not watch television all day — no woman would have time for that, anyway — needs about 2200 calories daily. One fact stands out, however, and that is that the average woman needs fewer calories per day than the average man. In other words, women are lucky as they don't have to eat so much of the energy foods in order to remain at their ideal weight as do men.

For people doing heavy work the energy expenditure will be much above the average. For instance, it is estimated that a woodcutter will need about 5500 calories daily. On the other hand, a man who sits at his desk from nine to five and watches television at night, uses up perhaps only 2100 calories per day.

The same amount of work performed may require a different amount

of calories in different people. Some are economical in their movements, while others spend a lot of energy just performing a simple
task.

The sensible reducer cuts down on foods which are not essential
for good nutrition, and continues to enjoy the foods which contribute
to his well-being. He minimises his intake of fats and carbohydrates,
while continuing to nourish himself with the healthy proteins, minerals
and vitamins. Protein foods satisfy the appetite, and instead of settling
in unwanted places, they spread throughout the body to nourish and
rejuvenate all the tissues.

Fats of course are the worst enemies of the reducer, as they supply
9·3 calories per gram against only 4·2 calories for the same amount of
carbohydrates or proteins. Therefore the person intent on losing
weight keeps his fat intake to a minimum. About one tablespoon of
fat is needed in the daily diet for lubrication purposes, but that is all.
Many foods contain some fat, so the quota is soon filled.

If you want to reduce, avoid fried foods. Frying increases the
calorie value of food items tremendously. For instance, if a boiled egg
represents 80 calories, then that same egg would have increased to
about 135 calories had it been fried in fat. The nutritional value
supplied by the egg remains the same, only the calorie count is ever
so much higher.

Use only very little butter or oil in cooking. Cut the fat off meat, and
grill your steak. Spread the butter or margarine much thinner on your
bread, and don't use mayonnaise with your salad. You can make your
own skim milk by siphoning from the bottle the cream which collects
on top of the milk. You drink the milk, and the cream goes to the cat
(but don't feed that poor animal too much either). Don't use cream
in your coffee, and avoid like the plague all dishes which are topped
off heavily with whipped cream.

Next in line for attention are the high-starch foods. Biscuits, cakes,
pastries, white bread, polished rice, noodles, spaghetti and macaroni
all help to pile on the pounds, and their intake therefore should be
sharply curtailed. A small piece of plain cake weighing only two
ounces means an addition of 200 calories to the diet. Surely this
allowance could have been spent in a better way.

Starch-reduced bread and biscuits don't make you slim, for there
is no slimming food as such. Weight for weight the caloric value of
starch-reduced bread is approximately the same as that of ordinary
bread, only there are more slices to the ounce. A slice of starch-
reduced bread contains fewer calories than an equally thick slice of
the normal bread variety.

In the average diet, much of the bodily iron requirement is supplied
by flour products. With a severe restriction of these foods, the iron
deficienty can be made up easily by the eating of other iron-containing

foods such as liver. The latter can also be consumed in the form of liverwurst.

Sugar means calories, and as is the case with starches, any excess is deposited in the adipose tissues. The sugar consumption, therefore, should be watched closely by the determined reducer. Refined sugar, chocolates, candies and sweet spreads in general do little more than decay the teeth and put on undesired weight. Preserves should be replaced by fresh fruit, and milkshakes by just plain milk. Better refreshments can be found than sweetened soft drinks and cordials.

Alcoholic drinks are high in calories, increase the appetite and destroy not only the B vitamins but also the reducer's good intentions. A 1 oz. nip of brandy or whisky is worth about 60 calories, a 3 oz. glass of dry sherry 90 calories, a 5 oz. glass of sweet table wine 100 calories, and a 10 oz. glass of beer 115 calories. A bottle of claret with dinner may mean more enjoyment but it also spells another 500 calories.

Tens of thousands of people refuse to eat various wholesome foods because these items are 'fattening'. Denying yourself adequate nourishment is not good for you. Being a sensible person, your reducing regime is a long-range programme based on the findings of science and the application of a little will-power. It is a matter of appreciating good health and of re-educating your appetite. Remember, it is all in the mind!

If you are planning a meal, include plenty of vegetables to supply goodness and bulk. Lettuce, tomatoes, celery, cabbage, cauliflower, Brussels sprouts, carrots, turnips and boiled onions can all be eaten freely by the reducer. Root vegetables contain a higher amount of carbohydrates than the green vegetables, but their calorie value is still low. Don't cover your lovely vegetables with a thick sauce. Instead of thickened soups, serve chicken broth without fat, or tomato bouillon.

When sitting down at the table, enjoy your meal but bravely refuse that second helping (a third helping is out of the question altogether, by golly!). Rich desserts undo all the sacrifices made during the whole day. Apple pie and cream may be what Mum used to spoil you with, but it is disastrous for your waistline. Just have a fresh apple without all the added calories. That will be healthier, and also much better for your teeth.

If you feel like eating something between meals, let it be a piece of fruit, or drink some fruit or vegetable juice. Unflavoured yoghurt is a good food, and it is filling.

Weigh yourself weekly. You don't have to lose pounds straight away, as long as you weigh a little less than the previous week. Even if you lose only 1 oz. per week, you are on the right track. It is better to lose two ounces each week than to lose two pounds during a week of misery and put it all back on again in a glorious weekend splurge. This will lead to mental frustration and physical exhaustion. A small but regular reduction in weight is much to be preferred. After all, if you lose two ounces each week, that would mean a yearly weight reduction of . . . let's see . . . six and a half pounds.

If you have not lost any weight at all at the end of a particular week, give yourself a lecture and eat a little less and exercise a little harder.

A wee over-indulgence now and then will do no permanent harm. We cannot always do exactly what we should do. Parties are attended, and business appointments have to be kept. Sometimes we just like to sin a little. No matter, you can do penance next day by minimising your food intake. You could miss a meal, or perhaps even have a complete fast. Having a fast one day a week would be a good idea, anyway. Just take some orange or grapefruit juice, and drink plenty of water. Such a short fast will make you feel good and wonderfully clean inside, and of course it will help you tremendously with your reducing programme. You could dedicate this one day fully to health and Yoga.

Lead a physically active life if you want to reduce. Movement counteracts the caloric effects of food. Besides, it improves the circulation and helps to keep the bloodvessels clear. Enjoy sports, and try to walk a few miles a day. Jogging would be better still. Instead of taking the lift, use the stairs. Of course, you must find a compromise here if you happen to work in the Empire State building. As with everything, common sense is the message.

8
The Royal Path

It is wonderful to be fit and healthy, and working to achieve perfect physical well-being means working towards a most useful goal. The practice of Yoga can be of help in realising this aim. To the Yogi, however, the practice of *Hatha* Yoga is only a preliminary to a much greater goal. Yoga teaches that conscious evolution is inherent in man, and that within his own lifetime man can attain a higher state of consciousness. Western psychology has made us familiar with the existence of a large and unknown region below the conscious mind which governs our actions. Yoga would agree with this concept, but also holds that there is another region of the mind, a zone above the everyday mind, which is called the superconscious mind. Whereas the subconscious mind is the seat of basic instincts and man there is close to the animal, the superconscious mind touches Infinity. All that is good and beautiful in human nature springs from the super-conscious mind. Through the practice of Yoga man can evolve to this higher stage of consciousness and attain the most felicitous condition of existence on earth.

That it is not necessary to excel in Hatha Yoga in order to progress further in Yoga can be gathered, for instance, from the attention paid to the physical aspect by Patanjali. This Indian sage, who is often called the 'Father of Yoga', lived about 300 B.C. He wrote the Yoga Sutras, the text book of mental Yoga. In this work Patanjali teaches that a complete Yoga programme consists of eight steps. The third step is Asana, or Yogic Posture. All the ancient master has to say on the subject is that a posture should be firm and comfortable. Hatha Yoga has its place, but there is no need to be a contortionist if you want to study and practise the higher aspects of Yoga.

Mental Yoga is called *Raja* (Royal) Yoga, and Patanjali's treatise makes a fascinating subject for study. The mind must be stilled, Patanjali says, if man is to become aware of his own true nature. The student must learn to be master over his thoughts and emotions. The mind can be made still be persistent efforts at restraining the mental activities and also by establishing an attitude of non-attachment to material things. So long as the student is attracted to worldly values he has no hope of establishing absolute control over his mind. Like the bird in a gilded cage, he will be held captive by his desires. Non-attachment, in Sanskrit called *vairagya*, is the foundation for progress in Yoga. *Vairagya* is not an end in itself but is a preparation for the achievement of the highest good. The final goal can only be reached

with the total annihilation of all selfish desires. Sense-objects themselves are not the cause of attachment. A particular object may
attract one person, repel another, and leave a third indifferent. Nor
are the sense-organs to blame. The cause of attachment lies in the
mind, which longs for a perpetuation of pleasurable experiences. The
student should be able to look at something and appreciate perhaps
its beauty and general usefulness, but he should not become emotion-
ally involved. He should not want to touch, taste, smell, hold, or
possess it. When he overcomes his likes and dislikes, he is no longer
afflicted by these emotional states.

Persistent efforts to restrain the various mental activities should be
made. The untrained mind is usually in turmoil, and as long as this
condition continues, the student will stay bound by his weaknesses
and remain a pitiful victim of circumstance. Often people act blindly,
not knowing the motives for their actions, nor realising the conse-
quences of their deeds. They follow the line of least resistance, seeking
pleasure and avoiding pain. If a person were to sit down and ask
himself at the end of the day how many of his actions were taken after
conscious deliberation, he would probably be lost for an answer. The
aspirant must question his motives and analyse his thoughts — a process of mind examining mind. He must look at the flow of ideas in
his mind objectively, and learn to detach himself from emotional
experiences. The quest for mastery over the mind will prove to be a
fascinating one. The student must break old habits and adopt a new
set of values. Sufferings will be met with patience, and adverse
circumstances will be regarded as opportunities for the exercise of
self-control. Complete mastery over the mind is established when the
aspirant can suspend all thought at any given moment and for any
desired duration of time. He will then be able to direct his thought at
will and by his own choice entertain only thoughts in conformity with
the Yoga creed.

Patanjali gives several directions on methods and attitudes. The
mind can be made calm by breathing exercises and by thoughts of a
selfless person. For calmness of mind an attitude must be adopted
of friendliness towards happiness, of compassion towards misery, of
gladness towards good and of indifference towards evil. Mental
purity is of the utmost importance, as impure thoughts result in misery
and ignorance (which is the generating cause of all misery). To
annihilate impure thoughts, contrary thoughts should be entertained.
All negative ideas should be substituted by positive thoughts. For
instance, as soon as the trainee finds himself thinking something
hateful, he should dismiss this thought immediately and dwell
instead upon a thought of love. Similarly, a pessimistic idea would be
replaced by an optimistic thought. All thoughts leading to oneness
are cultivated, and the rest are banished.

From mental purity arise cheerfulness, control over the senses, and the ability to concentrate. By the practice of the different stages of Yoga the impurities in the mind are destroyed, and the mind becomes a receptive vehicle for spiritual knowledge.

These are the eight stages of Yoga:—

1 Abstention (*yama*)
2 Observance (*niyama*)
3 Posture (*asana*)
4 Breath Control (*pranayama*)
5 Sense Withdrawal (*pratyahara*)
6 Concentration (*dharana*)
7 Meditation (*dhyana*)
8 Superconsciousness (*samadhi*)

Adherence to a high standard of ethics is required of the student intent on ultimate success in Yoga. Wearing a yellow robe or a flowing beard are only external criteria. The aspirant must lead an upright and moral life. The five abstentions are non-injury, truthfulness, non-theft, continence and non-greed. The five observances are purity, contentment, austerity, study and devotion to Divinity. The ideal is to maintain these precepts in all circumstances and at all times. Especially important is the principle of non-injury, called *ahimsa* in sanskrit. It demands of the aspirant a spirit of friendliness to all that lives. He should go through life bearing malice towards none, and love his neighbour as himself.

Controlled inhalation and exhalation make the mind fit for the practice of concentration. 'When the breath moves, the mind also moves', it is stated in an ancient Yoga classic. The breathing action is closely related to our mental activities. There are quite a few Yogic breathing exercises, but Patanjali does not list any of these. However, showing control over the breath by inhaling slowly and evenly, and exhaling in the same manner, is a most beneficial exercise.

In order to be able to concentrate fully, the messages from the senses should be disregarded. The mind must be isolated from the body and from the external world. The aspirant must learn to concentrate and be able to hold his mind steadily on the subject of concentration just as the rays of the sun are brought to a point of burning intensity by a magnifying glass. Concentration can be developed by the practice of mental exercises while concentration should also be applied to everything being done. Once he has the power of concentration, the aspirant is ready for meditation.

Whereas in concentration the subject can be anything, in Yogic meditation the idea pondered is always of a spiritual nature. The mind should be under such control that holding the subject of mediation in focus should require no effort at all. Scattered moments of insight will result.

In *samadhi* the mind is transcended, and the meditator achieves a new dimension of existence. He enters a state of spiritual ecstasy and absolute bliss. It is an experience beyond the range of the five senses, and beyond reasoning and intellect. All feeling of duality is permanently destroyed. The Yogi knows and feels in his innermost being that he is an integral part of the All.

If you have practised *Hatha* Yoga, you will have noticed the calming effect the postures and controlled breathing have on the mind. Adoption of a few of the attitudes and techniques of *Raja* Yoga can help you to gain some measure of control over your mind. For the attainment of poise, tranquillity and inner strength, the introspective system of psychology offered by Yoga has no parallel. If everyone lived according to the great principles of Yoga, dishonesty and hypocrisy would disappear. As man began to realise his fellow-man is of the same essence as himself, and that the human race is really one large family, hate and war would be replaced by universal love. There would be peace in the heart of men, and lasting peace would reign on earth.